FROM HERE TO PATERNITY

FROM HERE TO PATERNITY

THE DIARY OF A PREGNANT MAN

ANDREW CULLEN

ff

First published in 2006 by Fusion Press,
a division of Satin Publications Ltd
101 Southwark Street
London SE1 0JF
UK
info@visionpaperbacks.co.uk
www.visionpaperbacks.co.uk
Publisher: Sheena Dewan

A catalogue record for this book is available from the British Library.

ISBN-13: 978-1-905745-02-9
ISBN-10: 1-905745-02-8

2 4 6 8 10 9 7 5 3

Cover illustration: Andrew Cullen
Cover and text design by ok?design
Printed and bound in the UK by Creative Print and Design (Wales),
Ebbw Vale

CONTENTS

EPILOGUE   1

THE DIARY   5

INTRODUCTION   262

EPILOGUE

To breed or not to breed? That is the question.

Last week I went to a cinema, read a novel, walked up a mountain, ate in a restaurant with friends and had sex four times.

Why spoil it all by having children?

A lot of people seem to have children because they can't think of anything better to do. In many cases the primary qualification for parenthood is a lack of imagination.

Kate also has mixed feelings. Her grandmother once gave her this advice: 'Don't have any kids, they stop you living your life.'

I don't know if I am equipped to be a parent. I belong to a generation of adultescents that has turned self-indulgence into a religion. Children are relentlessly demanding and self-centred; in other words, they usurp our roles.

Over the years many of my friends, one way or another, have become mums and dads. It is nice to take the children off their parents' hands and play with them for five minutes. When they become excessively noisy or smelly, it is equally pleasing to hand them back.

I like children. It is parenthood that repels me. You are a slave to your child's needs. It pukes and poohs wantonly and leaves you to clean up the mess. It screams for attention and, when it has your attention, sometimes it carries on screaming. It can grant and withdraw affection with cruel whimfulness. It hits you. It throws things. You pick things up and it throws them again. If an adult treated you like this, it would be regarded as an abusive relationship; it would be grounds for divorce. They fuck you up, your kids.

Yet my friends with kids all say the same thing. 'It's worth it.'

Sometimes you have to make a decision: it's now or never. But with parenthood, the choice isn't that simple. It's now or later. Until one day I realised that I was in my 30s. How did that happen? I was as close to 50 as I was to 25. This was deeply depressing. Twenty-five feels like yesterday. So 50 is tomorrow. I'll be a pensioner the day after tomorrow. This time next week I'll be dead. We don't get much time between the womb and the tomb. Suddenly the choice has changed: it's now or soon.

Occasionally I stopped to consider the futures ahead of me, with or without children. Whenever I contemplated a lifetime of holidays and cinemas and possessions, the relentless consumption of goods and experiences, it left me feeling hollow. I'd like my life to be about something more substantial than the accumulation of CDs and holiday photos. I'm hoping that parenthood will be a way of living and giving at the same time.

We never actually said to each other that we were trying to get pregnant. As if putting it into words would put unnecessary pressure on us. We discussed the pros and cons without reaching a definite conclusion. One day, at a crucial moment, neither of us reached out for a condom.

Afterwards, Kate said: 'So are we not using condoms any more, then?'

'Apparently not.'

Human history is a succession of painful transitions. The industrial revolution of the 19th century, like the technological revolution we're living through now, impacted significantly on the way people lived and worked. Whether they wanted to or not, people had to adapt to profound changes in their daily lives. Many protested, but yielded in the end to overwhelming forces of change.

The history of an individual, like the history of a society, is also a sequence of uncomfortable transitions affecting one's sense of security and identity. No period of social upheaval has ever produced more intense emotions than the average adolescence. Even in adulthood, evolutionary and revolutionary pressures constantly challenge our search for emotional and material stability. Marriage seems to be a natural stage of evolution in most people's lives, whereas redundancy and divorce tend to be violent revolutions. We are continually adapting to new roles and new rules.

'You cross a one-way bridge when you have your first child. You can look back to where you have been, but you can never go back there,' says

Kate Figes in the first chapter of *Life After Birth*. Her book is described as 'the complete manual of the terrors, exhaustion and passionate emotions of the post-partum existence'. It is intelligent, insightful and well written. Except for this sentence: 'Men carry on living and working in the world in much the same way as they have always done, while women suddenly have cultural expectations of motherhood to live up to.'

On the contrary, men are also profoundly changed by the experience of becoming a parent. I have seen the evidence for this in the lives of my friends who are dads. Most of them have carried on working, but the vicissitudes of pregnancy and birth and childcare have altered their attitude to work, money, time, relationships, everything. Men suddenly have cultural expectations of fatherhood to live up to. I certainly didn't feel that I was going to carry on living and working in the world in much the same way as I have always done.

Pregnancy is a time of strange cravings. I suddenly acquired an insatiable appetite for books about pregnancy and birth. For us it was unknown territory. So I went to the bookshop for a guidebook.

Pregnancy manuals tend to concentrate on the biology and the practicalities. Any description of the man's role tends to be brief and superficial, accompanied by photos of a smiling man massaging a pregnant woman's back and looking implausibly cheerful considering he hasn't had sex for several months.

The social obligation to appear confident and self-assured creates an impossible ideal; people are disappointed in themselves for having natural feelings of insecurity and doubt. In the same way that society subjects us to impossible ideals of how we should look, it imposes unrealistic models of how we should feel. You are left doubting the validity of your own feelings. Am I feeling the right things? Is this what it's supposed to feel like?

It's fair to say that I didn't feel like the dads in the pregnancy books, relentlessly smiling and supportive, unafflicted by ambivalence or self-doubt.

Psychologists say that an individual's personality is an amalgamation of conflicting and competing impulses; we are 'a community of selves'. But the media presents a simplified version of human behaviour: the average newspaper or soap opera portrays human intentions as fixed and uncomplicated and describes events as a mechanical, logical narrative.

People's lives seem orderly and composed. A simple recounting of the facts – 'they met, they lived together, they got pregnant, they had a baby' – gives a false impression of implacable purposefulness and inevitability. Like an ocean that appears placid and flat from a distance, it's only when you look more closely that you see how choppy and stormy it is, with a tumult of life below its surface. Life stories, like all history, tend to omit the messy details for the sake of an artificial narrative clarity, an insistence on simple causes and effects that belies the complexity and confusion of real lives.

'How are you?' friends asked me during the pregnancy.

'Fine,' I always said. People who aren't pregnant don't really want a detailed description of your daily emotional upheavals.

This book is for those people who are interested in the messy details. It is unsuitable for inner children unless accompanied by an adult.

When we discovered that Kate was pregnant, I decided to write about what was happening to us. Some people adopt a policy of denial. I chose the opposite way and tried to pay attention. This is your life. You may as well take an interest.

It became a kind of travel book, an account of my journey from here to paternity. A diary seemed the least disingenuous literary form. The moment you start to structure your life into a coherent narrative with clear themes, you are telling a lie. The stories we tell naturally gravitate towards the dramatic moments of our lives; but most of our time is spent in the spaces in between. That's where we do most of our living and feeling. This diary is repetitive, whining and often contradictory. In other words, it is as true to life as I can make it.

'No one is boring who will tell the truth about himself,' said Quentin Crisp. I hope he's right.

THE DIARY

'The life of every man is a diary in which he means to write one story, and writes another; and his humblest hour is when he compares the volume as it is with that he would like to make it.' – J M Barrie

Sunday 29 September

So we might not be infertile after all. We were starting to wonder. We have been trying for four months. It hasn't always been a romantic or dignified process. Once or twice, Kate did a shoulder stand to help the sperm on its way.

Now her period is two and a half weeks late. Yesterday we bought a pregnancy-testing kit in Sainsbury's. The instruction leaflet said 'avoid excessive fluid intake before testing'. What does this mean? How much fluid intake is excessive? A cup of tea? We decided to wait until the morning.

In the early hours Kate jumped out of bed, went to the toilet and peed into a cup.

I shouted from under the duvet, 'I want to see!' So she came back into the bedroom with her cup of urine.

She placed the testing stick in the yellow liquid. I told her when 20 seconds had passed. She withdrew the stick from the urine and we stared. According to the leaflet, it would take about a minute for the results to appear.

There were two little windows on the stick. If a line appears in one window, it shows that the test has worked successfully. If a line appears in the other window, it indicates that you are pregnant.

A line appeared in one window almost immediately. 'That shows that the test has worked,' I said.

'No,' said Kate. 'That's the other window.'

I looked at the stick. I looked at the leaflet. I looked at the stick again. I said, 'Oh yeah. That means you're pregnant.'

We waited. Eventually a line appeared in the other window to confirm that the test was functioning properly.

I reached out and touched Kate, but she didn't move. I said, 'What are you waiting for?'

'For it to go away,' said Kate. She couldn't believe it was true. But the lines didn't go away. She smiled at me. It was a smile you can't fake. She was pleased.

'Oh shit,' I said, 'look where we live.'

Suddenly our one-bedroom flat seemed tiny. Where will we put the cot? When will we go to Peru? Do I want a baby? What will we call it? What if it's deformed? How am I going to make some money? These thoughts occupied about two seconds. They recurred throughout the day.

We know that you're supposed to keep the news to yourself for the first three months, so we agreed to keep it a secret.

Within an hour, I had told someone.

A newspaper photographer came to the house to take my photograph to accompany an article I've written for the *Independent*. Jack Hill sounded as if he had just got out of bed, yet he had managed to travel through morning fog all the way from Tooting on his motorbike. Making small talk while he clicked away, he asked what we were doing today. I found myself saying, 'Well, this morning we used a pregnancy test, and it was positive, so we're going to look at some books about babies.'

I said it matter-of-factly. I'm new at this. Maybe that's not how you're supposed to do it. The poor bloke looked as if he wasn't sure how to respond. After a couple of seconds he said, 'Congratulations …?'

The way he said it, it was partly a question. We assured him that we regarded this as good news. As he was leaving, he congratulated us again and shook my hand. Outside, the fog had disappeared; it was a beautiful day.

He was a stranger we'll never see again, so I felt able to tell him. I just wanted to share the good news. Kate forgave me.

After a trip to the library, we walked to Peckham Rye and spent the afternoon lying on the grass and reading in the sun. Kate was browsing through the *Complete Book of Pregnancy* and *Having Your First Baby after 30*. I was reading Miriam Stoppard's *Pregnancy & Birth Handbook*.

We learnt that one in five pregnancies end in miscarriage.

Miriam Stoppard assures me that it's natural to have mixed feelings about the pregnancy.

Despite everything – all the possible inconvenience and tragedy we're risking – we are happy. I can't lie to myself. I am pleased.

We agree that Thomas is a nice name for a boy, but its appeal is slightly diminished because my parents' cat is called Thomas.

We can't think of a girl's name. Kate suggests Lucy, but I used to know someone called Lucy and she has put me off the name. Every name reminds us of someone. We know too many people. Every prospective name for this pure innocent baby is tainted by association with the imperfections of real people.

The books are useful. They explain why Kate has had tender breasts. It's the progesterone preparing the glands for milk production.

One of the books says that 'a woman might experience a lower libido in the first stages of pregnancy'. That explains the past few weeks.

All the books mention the likelihood of mood swings. Sure enough, Kate was indicating that her mood had swung. There was a gleam in her eye. I haven't seen that gleam for a while. It was lovely sitting on the grass in the sunshine. But here was an opportunity not to be missed. We went home, walking quickly.

In romantic novels, the moment you conceive a child is invariably a blissful union. Maybe ours was. We can't remember the occasion. It was possibly the weekend we went to the Notting Hill Carnival. But the first time you make love after discovering that you're having a baby is also wonderful. Or maybe sex is always extra special when you haven't had it for three weeks.

Later in the afternoon we met friends. We managed not to tell them.

Monday 30 September

Today I walked through Dulwich Park. It was mostly populated by mothers, babies and toddlers. I was looking for signs of … I don't know … signs of what to expect. All the mothers in the pregnancy books are smiling, but the mothers in Dulwich Park aren't.

Kate phoned the Family Planning Clinic and told them she was pregnant. The woman said, 'And are you keeping it?'

'Yes, we are.'

Kate was told to contact her GP. The Family Planning Clinic is for people who are not planning to have a family.

'Is there no milk?' asked Kate when she came home from work.

I hadn't noticed. In my head I could hear Miriam Stoppard's voice: 'As your baby grows, so your calcium requirements increase – by week 25 they have more than doubled.'

I was busy. I didn't want to go to the shop. But this was the first test. I made myself sound more benevolent than I was feeling. I said, 'Do you want me to go to the corner shop and get some?'

'I want organic milk,' she said.

The corner shop doesn't have organic milk. 'Do you want me to go to Sainsbury's and get some?' My tone was slightly less benevolent.

'Yes.'

'Do you want anything else?'

'No. Oh yes, there is one thing you can get …'

Soon there were five things. Organic cereal bars containing nuts, kiwi fruit, orange juice, yogurt with active bio cultures, broccoli.

All evening Kate kept saying, 'I'm pregnant!' and 'You're going to be a dad!' She was just putting it into words to see if that made it seem more real.

Tuesday 1 October

We went to register the pregnancy with her GP. In the waiting room, she said, 'Are there any questions you want to ask the doctor?'

I said, 'What the hell do we do now?'

The waiting room has a television. This morning's debate on *Kilroy* was 'Do Children Need Two Parents?' To me it's obvious that children don't need two parents. They need about ten parents, just to allow a reasonable division of labour and a pattern of shift work that conforms to health and safety regulations. Unfortunately for parents, two is the most you can hope for.

One woman was telling Kilroy that her drug-taking and her clinical depression were caused by her parents' separation when she was nine. She was one of several adults telling Kilroy how much they were damaged by their childhood. It emphasises our new responsibilities.

The doctor summoned us. Kate told him, 'I've just had a positive pregnancy test.'

'Lovely, that's great,' said Dr Rajiv Patel. He seemed to mean it. I suppose a doctor never really knows what he is going to hear when a patient walks through the door. Having a baby is one of the few cheerful possibilities.

'Have you been taking folic acid?' he asked.

'Yes, for a month and a half,' said Kate, 'but not religiously.'

'Well, I hope you're taking it religiously now.'

He told us to make an antenatal appointment with the midwife who will discuss things with us in more detail. For example, where do we want to have the baby? We don't have to decide now. We have until Friday, when we see the midwife.

I'm having a baby at a peculiar time in my life. I've never been poorer. I have a low-income or no-income occupation. Parenthood wasn't one of my life's ambitions so my lack of financial qualifications for the role never seemed a problem. Now it is.

Playwrights aren't well paid, if they're paid at all. Apart from a few hundred pounds from newspaper articles, I haven't been paid for two years. Financial insecurity is a fact of life for a writer. But it shouldn't be a fact of life for a baby.

I have written a film script but so far, despite having Tim Roth and Rachel Weisz agree to play the leading roles, my producers, Stan and Ollie, haven't raised the money to make it. Then today, after five years of trying, my producer told me that the film is 100 per cent financed. Maybe everything's going to be fine after all.

It's hard to concentrate on work. It's hard to concentrate on anything.

Kate said tonight, 'It's scary. The changes in my body.' The main change so far is that she has a big smile on her face.

The pregnancy tester came with two sticks. This evening we used the second one to check the result of the first one. Kate crouched over the toilet. The instructions on the box say: 'Easy. Just hold the absorbent sampler in your urine stream for five seconds.' It isn't easy. Aiming is tricky. Having successfully avoided excessive fluid intake, Kate produced a dribble scarcely lasting the required five seconds. But it was enough. The blue line appeared in the square window. We are having a baby.

Kate said to me: 'You're going to be the father of my child.'

Already the pregnancy is changing what we are to each other. It is also changing what we are to ourselves. I'm feeling absurdly proud of myself, even though I haven't done much.

Wednesday 2 October
Kate mentioned it again. Something she read. 'One in five pregnancies ends in miscarriage.'

I tell her not to worry about this, not to think about it. But I think and worry about it.

One in five. If those were the odds on a horse in the Grand National, I might risk £5 on a bet. But we are investing our hearts and minds in this baby.

Despite the anxieties, we're quite enjoying being pregnant so far. Admittedly, it's only been three days.

It's true what they say. Pregnancy improves your skin and makes you glow with a new vitality. And that's just me. Kate is looking especially beautiful.

She keeps saying: 'We're having a baby! I can't believe it! Can you?'

It's no big deal in global terms. According to the World Health Organization, there are 100 million acts of sexual intercourse every day and 910,000 of them result in conception. But to us the event is momentous. It's a whole new world. This baby is one small step for mankind, one giant leap for us.

Thursday 3 October
So much for glowing with health and vitality. We both feel rough. I woke at 3 am and couldn't get back to sleep. I was thinking about money and death and roads not travelled.

Kate is finding it hard not to tell people. Last night she asked if I am also finding it difficult to keep the secret. I said no, not really. This is because I never see anyone. I work alone at home.

This morning I told someone. I've been having some knee pain so I had to go to the foot specialist in a local clinic. The woman told me that I have tight calf muscles and collapsing arches. I laughed. She asked what I was laughing at. I pointed to the poster on the wall. It was a grotesque picture of a crying baby. I said, 'We're having a baby and that poster kind of puts me off.'

She laughed as well.

She said, 'Yes, what to expect.'

I'm clearly not very good at keeping a secret. So far I have told a newspaper photographer and a podiatrist.

I like telling people. It's helping me get used to the idea.

On the way home I bought a book called *Having A Baby*.

According to *Having A Baby*, our baby's nervous system has started to develop, and this week our baby is forming a head. Its brain is developing, its heart is beating and there are small buds where its arms and legs are starting to grow. It has the beginnings of eyes and ears.

All the pregnancy books are adamant that alcohol and smoking are evil. Kate is concerned about the amount of alcohol that she drank at her friend's hen party several weekends ago. The books warn against binge drinking while pregnant. I have been telling her not to worry about it. Now I am worrying about it. But there's no point adding to her anxiety. I've decided not to raise the subject.

But this evening I found myself saying: 'So … how much did you drink?'

'Three glasses of champagne and a glass of white wine.'

'That's not much,' I said. I'm trying to say the right things, even though I'm not necessarily thinking them. 'It's not as bad as smoking. You didn't have any cigarettes, did you?'

'No.'

'That's fine, then. Let's not worry about it.'

Five minutes later she came up to me and hid her head in my chest. She said, 'I had one cigarette.'

Friday 4 October
Today we had our first antenatal appointment with the midwife at our GP's surgery. While we were waiting, we had time to examine the leaflets advertising various resources available to parents. One leaflet was promoting a weekend workshop for mothers. 'DO YOU WONDER WHERE YOUR LIFE HAS GONE? FEELING TRAPPED? SWAMPED? OVERWHELMED? DO YOU FEEL LOVE AND ANGER AT THE SAME TIME?'

After this bleak portrayal of parenthood, it seemed odd when the midwife greeted us by saying: 'Hello! First of all … congratulations!'

Fiona filled in a form detailing Kate's medical history.

Kate mentioned the cigarette that she had smoked in her third week of pregnancy. Fiona said, 'The baby won't mind about one cigarette.'

Kate told Fiona that she intends to breastfeed and she wants to have the baby in hospital rather than at home.

The disadvantage of giving birth in hospital is that it's likely that the midwife attending the birth will be a stranger. Kate would prefer to have someone she has met before, but the hospital will only arrange this if she is vulnerable: a teenage mother or a depressed mother or a drug-user.

Fiona took Kate's blood pressure. That was all.

Afterwards Kate was annoyed that Fiona hadn't even asked my name. I hadn't noticed.

Fiona has given us a pregnancy information pack. One of the booklets is called *Emma's Diary*, a fictional account of a pregnancy interspersed with adverts from Fisher Price, Johnson & Johnson, Sanatogen Pro-Natal, Tesco, Sainsbury's, Huggies, Persil, Babies R Us and 24 other companies. Some of these companies are kindly offering us free gifts. All they want are our registration details.

We are being targeted already. The examination from Tesco is more searching than the one from the midwife. The midwife might not be interested in the baby's father, but these companies want to know all about me. They want to know my occupation, the newspaper I read and if I have a credit card, a DVD, a dishwasher or a personal loan. They want to know the baby's due date, when we haven't even told our parents yet.

If you know the date of your last monthly period, you can work out the date your baby will be due. Kate's last period was on 18 August, so our baby is due on 25 May.

Kate was tired and grumpy today, although she would only admit to being tired. Her breasts were sore.

We cooked nice food and watched television. Rachel, one of the characters on *Friends*, is pregnant. In tonight's episode Rachel, Chandler and Monica watch a video of someone giving birth. They are all disgusted and horrified by the mother's ordeal. One of them asks, 'Have her eyes exploded?' Kate laughed uneasily.

When we're in the bedroom I say, 'Your breasts are bigger.'

'I know. If they're this big now, what will they be like in a few months?'

'It'll be the best Christmas ever.'

Saturday 5 October

I find myself noticing babies. Two parents of a newborn were eating at the pub. They didn't seem trapped, swamped or overwhelmed. Just knackered.

Kate has gone away for four days. She phoned from Yorkshire to say that she has told her friend Jenny about the pregnancy. We had agreed that she could. 'It's exciting talking to someone else about it.'

It is a hen weekend. A gang of women went to a restaurant this evening and spent the entire meal talking about babies. Kate resisted the temptation to announce that she is pregnant. Suddenly she has to lie to her friends. To explain why she can't drink alcohol or go for a hot spa at Harrogate Baths tomorrow, she has told everyone that she has an ear infection and is taking antibiotics.

Sunday 6 October   **Week 8**

Lots of children in Sainsbury's. I hope our child isn't fat. But that's the least of my fears. I heard on the radio today that 1 in 50 babies is born with some kind of defect.

Best not to think about it. Beyond ensuring that Kate is as healthy and happy as possible, there's not much we can do except hope our baby is one of the lucky ones. We are at the mercy of the gods.

Jenny phoned this evening to congratulate me. I congratulated her. She is about to go travelling around the world for six months – whereas we are embarking on seven months of vomiting and pelvic floor exercises.

Monday 7 October

One of the books says that red raspberry leaf tea taken during pregnancy, especially during the last three weeks, is supposed to 'tone' the womb, make contractions more effective, allow a faster, less painful birth and reduce bleeding. Apparently cows about to calf seek out raspberry leaves. That was today's big news. Oh, and the peace process is collapsing in Northern Ireland. Ours is not the only story in the world.

I have numbered the weeks on the calendar. This is week eight. Which means our baby is about to graduate from an embryo into a foetus. It feels like progress.

Tuesday 8 October

Kate is attending a conference near Manchester, so she spent last night at my parents' house in Warrington and caught the train back to London this evening. I met her in the street to help carry her bags. Her conversation was limited to 'I'm very tired' and 'My tummy hurts'.

She went straight to bed. Her tummy aches. We examined her abdomen for signs of a bulge. It's definitely there. It could be the baby, or it could just be the effects of one of my mum's meals. My mum and step-father go to a lot of effort when we visit. Every meal is the size of a Christmas dinner.

Kate has told three more people she is pregnant, all of them strangers, including the shop assistant in Marks & Spencer where Kate was looking for a bigger bra and a woman she sat next to on the Manchester–London train. This woman, who has three kids, has also read *Emma's Diary* and also finds Emma annoying. 'She's so healthy.'

Emma's fictional husband is presented as a model of understanding and selfless stoicism in the diary. 'Peter was a bit moody today. I think it's because we haven't made love for ages, but he says it's just that he's worried about me and how he's going to cope with fatherhood.' There is a photo of Peter. He doesn't look moody at all. Square-jawed, lightly tanned, casually smart, he is sitting (not slouching) on the sofa with his arm around Emma who is leaning against him. Looking at Peter makes you want to sit up straight. It's only a photograph but you can almost smell the aftershave. I would like to read Peter's diary to know what he's really thinking.

I said 'night night' to the baby through Kate's belly button.

Wednesday 9 October
My friend Nicola in Paris has had a baby boy. A card arrived announcing the birth of Marc. There's a photo of a sleeping baby with a big head. My first thought was, 'Cute.' My second thought was, 'How is that going to fit through Kate's vagina?'

I want to tell people the amazing thing that's happening to us.

At the same time, I dread telling people. Once it's out there, the news can't be withdrawn or controlled. Social intercourse is changed forever.

One reason we're not telling friends and family yet is to delay the clamour and the fuss that will inevitably follow the announcement. No doubt we are facing two decades of child-centred discourse. By keeping the news to ourselves, we are waiting for the pregnancy to become established, and we're also allowing ourselves a few more weeks of freedom from baby talk.

Thursday 10 October
I listened to a programme on Radio 4 about lack of sleep. A woman with three young children complained that she hasn't had a full night's sleep for four years.

I asked Kate if she has mixed feelings about being pregnant.

'I had doubts before I was pregnant,' she said, 'but now I just feel happy.'

She said she had 'a splitting headache'. According to the books you're allowed to take paracetamol but not aspirin. In the end she took neither.

Friday 11 October
Spoke to my film's producer on the phone this morning. 'Disaster!' said Ollie. An actor we wanted for our film, Dougray Scott, has accepted a more lucrative role in another movie. Without Dougray, we lose our finance. This means that my prospective earnings for the next six months are reduced to zero.

I went to a meeting in Soho House with my producers and the film's director, Sir Peter Hall.

Peter Hall explained that he'll have to accept offers to do other things because he can't afford not to work. He has already turned down theatre work to be available for our project. 'Unless you can guarantee that the film is financed?'

One of my producers, Ivan, said: 'I expect the finance to be forthcoming, but nothing is guaranteed. As you know, there's many a slip. I've made twenty-five films and what I've learnt is that there's never a moment where you open the champagne.'

This made me laugh. I remember Ollie opening a bottle of champagne six years ago, shortly after we started this project. That was the first time that the film was '100 per cent financed'.

Even though Peter Hall's decision to withdraw from the project is utterly sensible and reasonable, he seemed to be on the verge of talking himself out of it. But the producers made no effort to encourage him. What Peter Hall doesn't know is that they have already been planning to replace him with another director who is younger and 'hipper'. Someone who, they think, is more attractive to film investors.

Later, when I told my agent, Laura, about this subterfuge, she was disgusted but not surprised: 'The film business is ageist and doesn't respect talent.'

In one morning we've lost our actor, our director and our finance.

I was tempted to tell Peter Hall that I'm having a baby. The last time I met him, we discussed the script all morning and then went to an Indian restaurant. While waiting for lunch to arrive, we made small talk about films and plays.

Out of the blue, Sir Peter Hall (former director of the Royal Shakespeare Company, successor to Olivier as director of the National Theatre, knighted in 1977) said: 'Have you got kids?'

'No.'

'That's the best thing,' he said. 'I recommend it.'

What I didn't know then was that Kate was already pregnant. Today I almost told him. But in the end I didn't mention it. I don't want the film producers to hear about it; I don't want their fake interest.

Back home, Kate asked why I was so glum.

I don't really know. It's not only the disappointment about the film. I've got used to that. It's also the parenthood thing. The awareness that a lot of choices, which theoretically were available to me, no longer are. I feel hemmed in. Trapped.

Kate said she has thought of another boy's name she likes. 'Max.'

I pulled a face. 'Everyone called Max is obnoxious. Max Hastings. Max Clifford. Max Headroom.'

'All right.' I seem to have talked her out of that one.

Then I remembered. 'I've thought of a girl's name I like.'

'What?'

'The name I like is _____.'

'Oh, I like _____.'

So _____ is a possibility.

Saturday 12 October

This morning we tried to have sex for the first time in a while. Kate's breasts are too sore to be touched or kissed, which is frustrating for both of us. We tried lying on our sides. But there was always a limb in the way. In the end we gave up, concluding that sex in this position will only be possible if we chop off one of our legs. The books say that sex during pregnancy is possible if you're patient and keep your sense of humour. I like to think that I have a sense of humour, but even Groucho Marx couldn't have sex in this position.

We went to see a play at the Tricycle Theatre with two friends. Afterwards, walking along a street in Kilburn, we saw a billboard poster: 'SMOKING DURING PREGNANCY AND SECOND-HAND SMOKE CAUSE HALF THE NUMBER OF COT DEATHS.' We bought a mountain of food from an Indian restaurant and took it to our friends' flat in Tufnell Park. After the meal they lit up cigarettes. It was hard not to hate them.

Sunday 13 October   Week 9

It hasn't rained for five weeks. Today was dark and wet. We stayed in bed, chatting pleasantly until Kate said, 'I think we should move house.'

A headline in the newspaper last week said that the average London house costs £200,000. Our one-bedroom flat in Peckham comprises the upper storey of a small terraced house in a street which, according to the 1890 census, used to be inhabited by candle-makers and domestic servants. Even this place, when we obtained a 95 per cent mortgage for it 18 months ago, thanks to a loan from Kate's mum, cost £112,000.

'I'd love to move to a bigger place,' I said, 'but let's wait and see.'

Later, she was reading about her pelvic floor muscles.

'I have to do my pelvic floor exercises while your penis is inside me,' she said.

'Really?'

'It's in the book.'

'Was the book written by a man?'

According to the book, it's my job to tell her how hard she is squeezing. I said, 'I'm happy to do anything I can to help.'

The nesting instinct seems to have emerged prematurely. Kate started putting up new curtains in the bedroom. While I was talking to a friend on the phone, she started sawing the curtain pole.

After a while she announced: 'I've cut the curtain pole too short.'

I found this irritating. 'Why are you doing this now?'

'If I don't, nothing gets done.'

I found this even more irritating. I started to list all the improvements I've made to our home. This list was shorter than I'd anticipated, but I waved my arms to suggest that I could continue indefinitely. 'Anyway, why didn't you ask me to help?'

'Why didn't you offer?'

'Because I'm doing other things. You're working to your own agenda. OK, let's make a list,' I heard myself shouting. 'What things do you want done?'

'Don't.' Tears were coming into her eyes.

This was the moment for me to stop. But I carried on. I was shouting. 'How am I going to get any work done when there's no fucking space and there's a fucking baby in the corner?'

'Don't.' She turned away. Now she was crying properly.

Ashamed, I stopped shouting. 'I'm sorry.'

'You said "*fucking baby*".'

She's right, I did use those words. I didn't mean them to sound so ugly. 'I'm sorry.' I rubbed her tummy. 'And I'm saying sorry to the baby.'

'You've never shouted at me before.'

'I know. I promise to try never to shout again. We mustn't let new pressures turn us into people who argue.'

'No.'

'We're having a baby. That's a wonderful thing. We mustn't forget that.'

'Yeah.'

'Let's make a list of things we want to do.'

'I've made a list.'

'Have you? Oh right.'

She showed me a list that she made back in August.

Monday 14 October

Didn't sleep very well. I never used to worry about money like this.

Stupidly, I have done a lot of unpaid work on the film script. My income last year was zero. I haven't even bought myself a pair of socks for two years. The baby will need socks. And nappies. And food.

In the evening, there was news about our actor. It seems that his other movie won't start filming until April. So he might be available for our film after all. We'll find out in the next few days if the financial investors, the bank, the film distributors and the tax fund are compatible. There's still hope.

I'm reminded of the line spoken by John Cleese in the film *Clockwise*: 'It's not the despair that gets me, it's the hope.'

There's no business like show business. Thank God. It's a ridiculous industry. My script is about life inside an English prison. Depending on who provides the money, we will have to film in the Isle of Man or Canada or Germany. If we use Canadian funding, 75 per cent of the actors will have to be Canadian. Originally the script was a challenging but heart-warming true story about a professional criminal, Norman, who decided to go straight when he was released from jail after 27 years. Three years into the project, I discovered that Norman wasn't as straight as I'd been told. He was carrying a gun and delivering cocaine for one of the criminal gangs operating in North London. My producers knew this for at least a year before they bothered to tell me. When I was researching the script, I visited prisons and encountered con men, heavy drug-users and men with strange sexual habits. That turned out to be ideal preparation for working in the film business.

I was naïve to trust these people. When I told my mate Tom about this, he told me not to castigate myself. He said, 'What's so terrible about being naïve? I have embraced naïvety as a lifestyle choice. I am often guilty of behaving as if the world is the kind of place I want it to be: somewhere characterised by trust, respect and fair-mindedness. I know these traits aren't universal, but unless we live as if they are, we lose them altogether.'

Kate had an early night. For me, going to bed is less tempting than it used to be. These days, we just sleep. I worked until 2 am.

Tuesday 15 October

Tonight we discussed what we'll do if the ultrasound scan in November reveals that our baby has Down's syndrome. We have mixed feelings. If the scan shows that our child will be disabled, we'll have the option of killing the foetus. This seems unimaginably cruel. We already talk to the foetus through Kate's tummy. In theory, I'm in favour of a woman's right to an abortion. But now it isn't just theory. We don't really know what we'd do. We hope it's a decision we won't have to make.

Kate contemplated the bulge in her tummy. We're still not sure if that's the baby showing or if she has eaten too many biscuits.

I kissed her belly. Kate complained, 'I can't kiss the baby like that.'

'No, but you're holding it and carrying it round.'

'Are you envious?'

'No.'

I know that childbirth is supposed to be a transcendent experience, but it's one that I'm happy to forgo.

Worked until 2 am again.

I keep thinking about all the things we won't be able to do because we have a baby. I'm sure there are many compensating pleasures, but what are they?

Wednesday 16 October

The books say that a baby's movements are undetectable until weeks 18 to 22. We are only in week nine but Kate is concerned that she 'can't feel anything in there'. She looks frightened. I tell her not to worry.

'My breasts aren't sore any more.'

'Good. They're not meant to be sore for the entire pregnancy. People have different symptoms. Like … you've not had any morning sickness, have you?'

'They say that people who have morning sickness have less chance of a miscarriage.'

'Who says that? I've never heard anyone say that.'

'What if it's dead in there?'

'Lovey, everything's fine.'

These first weeks are difficult. The baby is an abstraction. How do we really know we're having a baby? All we've done is pee on a stick. During this pregnant pause, it is like waiting for the guests to arrive at your party. We have too much time to think about all the things that can go wrong. Or if the guest of honour will turn up.

Thursday 17 October

News from Warrington. My cousin has given birth to a girl. The baby's name is _____. Does this mean we have to abandon our favourite girl's name? I don't think so. Kate suggested Theresa instead but I quickly squashed that idea. There's a Tory MP called Theresa. She has ruined the name for me.

My cousin's husband has been studying for exams so they sent their baby to stay at the grandparents' house for a week so Dad could do some studying. I hear stories like this and wonder what we're in for.

Working at home, I waste a lot of time. I am ingenious at distracting myself. The imminent arrival of a baby has made me drift less, but not much.

I am worried that I won't be able to write at all when I'm sharing the flat with a baby. For a writer – according to Cyril Connolly – 'there is no more sombre enemy than the pram in the hall'.

Some writers seem to cope. On the radio recently I heard J G Ballard saying he never has trouble writing once he has sent the kids off to sleep or off to school; he just needs to encourage the creative juices by changing his state of consciousness, and he does this with a double whisky.

I once asked Alan Bleasdale how he managed to be so prolific in his 30s. He said, 'I had three kids.'

Most encouraging of all is Anne Tyler, an American novelist, who says this in an essay about writing and parenthood:

My Iranian cousin has just had a baby: she sits home now and cries a lot. She was working on her master's degree and is used to being out in the world more. 'Never mind,' I tell her, 'you'll soon be out again. This stage doesn't last long.' 'How long?' she asks. 'Oh ... three years, if you just have the one.' 'Three years!' I can see she's appalled. What I'm trying to say to her is that it's worth it. It seems to me that since I've had children, I've grown richer and deeper. They may have slowed down my writing for a while, but when I did write, I had more of a self to speak from. After all, who else in the world do you have to love, no matter what? Who else can you absolutely not give up on? My life seems more intricate. Also more dangerous.

Friday 18 October

Kate hasn't had much of an appetite for the past couple of days. Today at work she was eating celery for lunch because she didn't fancy the cheese sandwich she'd made. One of her colleagues noticed this and said, 'Celery!' She felt obliged to justify herself. 'I can't eat my sandwich. This is all I feel like eating.'

'Are you pregnant?'

'Pregnant!?' she said, and tried to laugh it off.

'You've gone all red.'

Even her baggy trousers are starting to feel tight. It's time to go shopping.

Saturday 19 October

I'm working long hours while I still can. In some ways, pregnancy has the same effect as a terminal disease; it makes you value every day you've got left. Last night I worked until 3 am. Five hours later, I was roused from a deep sleep by Kate's hand wandering across my groin.

I was so tired, not many things could have woken me, but this was one of them. Her libido had returned. I pretended to be asleep for a while longer so that she would continue what she was doing. Then I turned over and we began to make love. After a few minutes, she seemed to lose interest in the erotic aspect of proceedings. 'Can you feel that?' she said. She was squeezing my penis with her pelvic floor muscles. 'Yes, slightly.' 'Can you feel this?' 'Yes, that's a bit stronger.' Our lovemaking had turned into pelvic floor exercises. When she had finished, I turned over and went back to sleep.

We went to Richmond, strolled beside the Thames and climbed the hill to Richmond Park. We visited Henry VIII's Mound where the trees have been sculpted to allow a clear view across London to St Paul's Cathedral. We had supper at a friend's house in Raynes Park. Kate asked for a pint of milk to drink with the meal.

Terry said, 'Milk? Is there something you haven't told me?'

'No,' I said, 'she always drinks a lot of milk. She's funny like that.'

After supper, we all went to a birthday party in Wimbledon. People were smoking. We left early. We stood in the street saying goodnight to Terry. He said to Kate, 'You didn't drink any alcohol, did you?'

It's getting harder to keep the secret.

Sunday 20 October   **Week** 10

We've had an email from Ava, a friend in New Zealand. She is pregnant. She is only in the eighth week but she seems keen to tell everyone already. She sounds ecstatic. 'Due next June so it's too early to feel anything yet except excited … I'm very happy … this is what I want right now.'

I can't help comparing her undiluted joy with our cocktail of feelings. Kate says she hopes that she'll start to feel more wholeheartedly excited after the first scan. 'Right now it doesn't seem real.'

In the absence of anything to do, we keep finding things to worry about. I read today that 'smoking or inhaling other people's smoke in the first three weeks of pregnancy can cause cleft lip and palate'. That's something I dread.

A grey wet day. On BBC1 we watched a programme about Michael Palin travelling across the Sahara. This revived my wanderlust. I am starting to feel trapped by our baby, even though it hasn't been born yet.

I asked Kate, 'What do you think life will be like when the baby arrives?'

'I don't know,' she said. 'I haven't thought about it.'

'Shouldn't we have thought about it before we decided to have one?'

'I'm worried that you'll be frustrated.'

'So am I,' I replied unhelpfully.

We discussed various options. Can we afford to buy a larger flat? Should we rent somewhere? Should she work part-time? There are a thousand questions and no immediate answers. We concluded that things will work out.

As she was undressing for bed, I couldn't help noticing.

'Look at your breasts,' I said. 'What a shame I'm not allowed near them.'

'You will be soon.'

'When?'

'I don't know.'

I worked till 2 am. When I went to bed, Kate was awake.

'Can't sleep. I'm worried.'

'About what?'

'About us.'

'Sweetie, please don't worry, because I love you very, very, very much.'

We went to sleep.

Monday 21 October

At work, Kate sits at her desk with her button undone and her zip halfway down because her trousers are so tight. She is concerned that her jumper isn't long enough and someone will notice.

Kate decided to tell her mother, who lives in France, that she is pregnant. So she phoned. But her mum wasn't there.

We sat on the sofa and ended up talking about sex, fidelity and the future.

I promised that I would try my best to be faithful for the rest of our lives. This was the wrong thing to say.

'What do you mean, *try*?'

I was just being realistic. But this wasn't the moment for a philosophical approach. In the end I promised that I definitely will be faithful for the rest of our lives.

As Kate pointed out, the cost of failure has just gone up. If either one of us were unfaithful, we'd be betraying our child as well.

Tuesday 22 October

Loving someone doesn't stop you noticing other people's attractiveness, whatever the love songs say. 'I only have eyes for you,' sang Frank Sinatra. But he was married four times.

I've been thinking about the infidelity issue. Kate and I have been together for three and a half years and living together for eighteen months. We have often told each other that we want to stay together for the rest of our lives. But a baby is a new level of commitment. Now we're stuck with each other. The relationship feels different. Before, it was a choice; now it's an obligation.

It's like … er … you can happily sit in a room for hours, but if someone tells you to sit in a room for hours, suddenly it can feel like a prison. Even though it's the same room.

I love Kate. You know it's love when you feel lucky to have that person in your life. I feel very lucky.

If I were ever unfaithful, I'd hate myself even if I got away with it. I don't think two and a half minutes of pleasure is worth a lifetime of self-loathing.

But who can say what will happen? It's easy to be virtuous when you're happy and sober.

A few of my married friends – men and women – are having affairs. I know a man who pretends to play football every Sunday morning. He gets a friend in the football team to rub his shorts and shirt in the mud so he can give them to his wife to wash.

I don't want to live like that.

I could say, with hand on heart, that I never look at other women. But it would be a lie. Of course I look at them. Every day I see people I'd like to fuck and people I'd like to punch. But we're not children, unable to control every surge of emotion. We can't choose how we feel, but we can choose how we behave. We should at least try to. Even my happily married friends admit that they are occasionally distracted by some of the beautiful men and women in this city. So I feel consoled that I am not the only one who feels an occasional pang of regret for lost excitements; forgone but not forgotten. Married people will never again experience the pleasure of a First Kiss. We are limited to sex with one person for the rest of our lives. And even that isn't guaranteed.

If I'm ever tempted to be unfaithful, I have friends to remind me of the damage it can do. My mate Chris has three girlfriends at the moment, as well as someone he has phone-sex with. He meets women through work or through the personal ads in the *Guardian*. He once flew to Washington DC just to have sex with someone he'd met in an internet chat room. At the time, he was still living with his wife and four kids. His wife threw him out when she discovered his addiction to fucking other women. Ironically, Chris is a relationship counsellor.

Most of all, I think my father had a big influence on me. He is a role model. He is the kind of man, the kind of husband and the kind of father that I'd hate to be.

Wednesday 23 October
This morning Kate phoned me from work, asking me to buy a cheese and tomato pizza for her supper.

I went to see Caryl Churchill's latest play at the Royal Court. It's about a father whose son is cloned 20 times. It's a clever idea, but the play was barely more than an hour long. Instead of building to a climax, it just seemed to stop, as if they'd lost the last 30 pages.

When I got home, Kate told me that we will have to buy some earplugs. She'd watched a TV documentary which mentioned that a crying baby is as noisy as a pneumatic drill. Apparently the baby and the drill attain the same decibel levels.

Kate has been feeling queasy for a few days. She didn't fancy the cheese and tomato pizza after all, and ate less than half of it.

She is impatient for the first ultrasound examination, which is three weeks away. She wants confirmation that the baby is really there and that it's all right. She mentioned it again tonight. 'I wish it was time for the scan.'

I said, 'Lovey, we're having a baby. It takes nine months. Even for you. We can't rush things. Let's try and enjoy it.'

In a way I welcome her irrational fears because they distract attention from mine. And they give me a role, something useful to do. It's my job to be a calm and wise presence. This is a challenge, but I'm trying my best. I kissed her belly and she seemed to like that.

She is hypersensitive to smells at the moment. She was repelled by my pizza breath, even though I'd only eaten one slice.

Later she said sorry and gave me a kiss. But she wiped her mouth afterwards.

Thursday 24 October
Despite feeling queasy, Kate went to an antenatal aquarobics session in the local swimming pool. She says she enjoyed it, apart from when she felt some vomit rise into her mouth. Luckily she managed to swallow it.

I'm learning something new every day. What I've learnt today is never go to a public swimming pool after an antenatal class – you don't know what might be floating in the water.

Friday 25 October

I have started reading *A Good Enough Dad*, the actor Nigel Planer's account of becoming a father for the first time.

He says this: 'You have to be mad to have children. The less you know about what it will really be like, the better, otherwise no one would ever do it.' I haven't yet got to the bit where he says that, despite everything, it's worth it. I hope there is a bit like that.

I made an impulse purchase in W H Smith. I bought a magazine called *Practical Parenting*. When I went to pay for it, the friendly young woman behind the counter said, 'Are you having a baby?' As if I might just be buying it out of general interest.

When I was ten years old, I used to read every word on every page of a football magazine called *Shoot!* Now I am reading *Practical Parenting* with the same eagerness. Three weeks ago, apparently, our baby was the size of a baked bean. Now it is already the size of a chocolate-chip cookie.

I paid close attention to an article claiming to tell me everything I need to know about sex during pregnancy. In fact, this article failed to tell me the one thing I really want to know: will there be any?

A taxi took us to Dulwich where we had supper with friends. Kate told them that she can't drink alcohol because she is pregnant. Everyone said 'congratulations' without seeming particularly impressed by the news. Perhaps we were wrong to expect two gay men and a mother of three to share our sense of awe and excitement.

I asked the mother of three for any parenting tips. She said that her first baby got into the habit of falling asleep only when her parents were with her; consequently it was two and a half years before she would go to sleep without at least one of her parents being present. With her second child they 'maintained clearer boundaries' and that made life easier. That's her top tip. I've added it to everything else I've heard and read. It gives me a comforting illusion that I'll know what to do when the time comes.

At home, Kate had her daily moment of panic. 'What if something's wrong?'

I assured her confidently that everything is OK. I said, 'I love you very much. We're having a baby! I'm very happy.'

A good day. I said the right things. I felt the right things.

Saturday 26 October
Kate phoned her mum and told her that she's pregnant. Her mum's first response was, 'Do you want to be?'

'Yes,' said Kate. She thought her mum seemed pleased.

I think that one of my main duties during the pregnancy is not to whinge. But I keep failing. Every day brings a dreadful realisation. It seems obvious that, when we have kids, we won't be able to travel anywhere. 'Oh God,' I whined this morning, 'and if we ever do go on holiday, we can only go during school holidays, when everyone else is on holiday.'

My whining doesn't help Kate, of course. It would be better for her if I were the strong silent type. Unfortunately, I seem to be the weak talkative type.

We went to Tate Modern to see a giant sculpture by Anish Kapoor. A friend came with us and he was keen to go somewhere afterwards. It was Saturday evening in one of the world's great cities. But all Kate wanted to do was go home and lie on the sofa while I stroked her hair. So that's what we did. It's a 24-hour city. But we're 16-hour people.

'I'm sorry I'm so tired,' she keeps saying.

Sunday 27 October   Week 11
Gale-force winds. Kate walked behind me, using me as a windbreak.

There's a large Mothercare on Rye Lane in Peckham. I've walked past it a thousand times without noticing it. Until today. We'd only been inside for two minutes and I was just trying to recover from the price of cots when Kate said, 'Let's go. I'm feeling superstitious about being here.' So we had to leave.

At home, she felt very queasy. She said that her hands were trembling. 'I thought I was going to faint. It was scary.'

Monday 28 October
Depressed and worried about the film today. Other people's greed is preventing progress. One Canadian producer is demanding a fee of £70,000 just to introduce us to an investor. He wants £70,000 for making one phone call.

I went to Soho House to meet my producers and the film's new director, Mike Barker. The toilets have been refurbished; all the flat surfaces are now slanted to deter cocaine-sniffers.

Mike Barker told a story about the stresses of parenthood. One day his wife, in the middle of a dispute with their three-year-old daughter, shouted, 'Get her out of here or I'll smash her head!' Mike tried to assure the sobbing three-year-old that Mummy didn't mean it.

Mike said to me, 'Have you got kids?'

Nobody has asked me this question since I've known Kate is pregnant. I wasn't ready for it. I said: 'Er ... y ... n ... n-n-no, no.'

'You stuttered a bit there,' said Mike.

'I swear I haven't got any kids.'

I'm not going to tell these people about the baby.

Some conversations with Kate this evening:

'I'm worried.'

'What are you worried about?'

'I can't feel anything.'

I showed her the section in the magazine explaining that a pregnant woman can't feel the baby's movements until weeks 18–22.

Later she said, 'I think I might have twins.'

'What makes you think that?'

'I just think I'm quite big.'

One minute she thinks nothing's there, and the next minute she thinks it's twins.

'Look at my cleavage!'

'I know.'

Tuesday 29 October

I'm working my way through *Practical Parenting* magazine, which is a tragicomic epic to rival anything by Dickens or Dostoevsky. It has articles such as 'New Look Lego' next to 'My Pregnancy Put Me in a Wheelchair'.

When Kate came home from work, almost the first thing she said was: 'I had a really horny dream last night.'

'And you didn't wake me up?'

'You were fast asleep.'

'You have permission to wake me up.'

Actually, I'm getting used to not having sex. The nightly peaks of hope and troughs of disappointment gradually became less extreme; there were whole hours when I didn't think about it; now the notion of sex doesn't occur to me at all. I seem to have forgotten that it exists.

When I talk to the baby through her stomach, Kate uses a particular voice for the baby's replies. Now she has learnt a new tactic. She asks for things using the baby's voice. Tonight in bed the baby asked for a glass of water. I felt compelled to obey.

Wednesday 30 October

A friend of a friend is dying of cancer. Some years ago his sister died of leukaemia. Now the parents are about to watch another child suffer a cruel premature death.

I've been watching the news with a different perspective. A fourteen-year-old girl was raped; three young children were killed by falling trees in stormy weather; numerous young people were killed by a bomb in Bali.

I'm realising that, when you're a parent, there's no time when you can stop worrying.

We watched a documentary about human instinct. It mentioned that women are more likely to be unfaithful during ovulation and claimed that one in ten men are unknowingly raising children without being the genetic parent. Kate turned to me and said, 'I promise you that you are the father of my child.'

There were football results on the television news. When I saw that Liverpool had lost, I automatically said, 'Fucking hell!'

'You won't be able to say "fucking" when the baby's here,' said Kate.

She stroked her tummy and said, 'I'm hairier.'

Thursday 31 October

We made love this morning. It came as a surprise to both of us. Possibly to all three of us, I don't know. It's good to know that everything's still working.

It's important that we don't become so baby-focused that we forget each other.

Friday 1 November

I've finished reading *A Good Enough Dad*. I became quite fond of Nigel Planer's family. His son, Stanley, says things like 'Daddy, a monster's eaten my holiday.' 'Flowers don't have bosoms, do they?' 'How will we see with the dark on?'

I looked on the internet to see if Nigel Planer has written any other books about fatherhood and was immensely sad to discover that he has separated from his wife and child. He has a baby son with his new wife. Twelve-year-old Stanley lives abroad with his mother.

Sometimes I look at my friends with children and feel encouraged; some complain more than others, some drink more than others, but everyone seems to cope. Then I remember how many divorces and separations there are among them.

If I just look at people I know, I can count 17 divorces. I can think of three friends whose relationships are disintegrating. They all have children. Kate's parents are divorced. In the UK, the average lifetime of a marriage is nine years.

I remember reading about the American soldiers who stormed Omaha beach in World War II. The first men to jump off the boats and run towards the German machine guns were exceptionally brave. But the men who followed them in the second wave were said to be even braver, because they went through with it despite seeing what had happened to the men who went first.

I have a similar feeling about relationships. People who go through with it, knowing the fate of those who have tried it before, should get a medal.

Saturday 2 November
Friends were coming round for lunch. We had to hide all the pregnancy books. This involved checking every room. *Practical Pregnancy* was in the loo, *The Social Baby* was in the kitchen. Six other books were scattered around the living room.

I went to the National Portrait Gallery to see Humphrey Spender talking about his work as a photographer for the *Daily Mirror* and *Picture Post* in the 1930s and 1940s. Amazing to see a man who witnessed the rise of Nazism and who was a friend of Isherwood and Auden. Now aged 92, he seemed robust and energetic. I tend to regard old age as a bitter battle against decay and dementia, based on the experiences of the grandmothers I know. All the grandads are dead. But Humphrey Spender has restored my faith in the possibility of resilience.

Having a baby makes me want to live as long as possible. Longevity might seem a natural ambition, regardless of whether or not you have children. But I can imagine circumstances that make living more trouble than it's worth. Some illnesses are so cruel they amount to torture. Being a parent is making me more fearful of that kind of eventuality. I feel as if I have a greater investment in the world, a reason to hang around as long as I can.

Later, Kate and I walked to Piccadilly to spend a couple of hours in Waterstone's. One of life's great pleasures is dawdling in a bookshop. Today we spent the whole time in Pregnancy and Childcare. I found some useful tips in a book called *The Parent's Survival Handbook*: 'When anyone asks you how your baby is, they actually only want an answer that lasts up to one minute'; 'If you must show pictures, limit yourself to two. Break the one minute/two picture rule and you run the risk of losing all your friends.'

There was a girl, aged about eight, sitting on one of the sofas. She was reading a book with a huge grin on her face. That's one thing I love about kids. They retain a capacity for joy, something that most adults seem to have lost.

Although I worry that parental duties will deprive us of some of life's pleasures, on the whole I am pleased that we have conceived sooner rather than later. The earlier in life you have kids, the longer you will have the pleasure of their company.

On the other hand, you don't know what kind of person they're going to be. One of my schoolmates killed his parents with an axe. They worked in the nuclear power industry and he claimed that he had killed them for 'ecological' reasons. Now he lives in a special hospital.

Parenthood is the ultimate blind date. It is a blind marriage.

Sunday 3 November   Week 12

Kate got up early and had breakfast. Later she came back to bed with no clothes on. 'For a cuddle.' We have a sex life again, although she has given me clear instructions: 'You can kiss my breasts but not the nipples.'

Sex during pregnancy is not impossible, but it's like trying to arrange a peace settlement in the Middle East; it only follows a series of delicate negotiations and territorial prohibitions so that both sides feel their needs are respected.

For lunch we went to Drew and Julia's house. By week 12, the risk of miscarriage is much reduced, so we were wondering whether to tell them that we're having a baby. I said to Kate, 'What's your instinct?'

'It seems easier to tell them. What's your instinct?'

'To leave it up to you.'

She told them. They have two kids, so they had plenty of stories.

The most disturbing thing for Julia in hospital was the sound of women screaming in other rooms.

Drew told us about their antenatal class. Everyone sat on chairs or cushions and introduced himself or herself. One man, sitting on a chair and wearing a woolly jumper with a picture of a dog on it, announced that he was a dog-trainer. His wife was sitting on a cushion at his feet. When she did well with the gas-and-air apparatus, he patted her on the head.

Drew told us what will happen to our social life. At first we'll hang out with those of our friends who have kids; then we'll end up hanging out with the parents of our kids' friends. So the old adage – you're stuck with your family but you can choose your friends – is untrue. Your family chooses your friends.

Monday 4 November

Kate has been feeling less nauseous and tired in recent days. We both feel calmer about the idea of having a baby, sometimes for minutes at a time.

Last year we spent a month in Nepal. As a way of making conversation, people often ask us if we're planning any more big trips. A friend asked me this today. The question provoked a pang of regret for a lost way of living. Parenthood is a senseless waste of a lifestyle.

I must stop thinking of children as a form of handicap.

Kate said tonight, 'I felt a couple of twinges. Needle pains. There.' She pointed to the right side of her stomach. 'I don't know what it is.'

'Just your stomach getting used to stretching,' I said reassuringly, as if I'm an expert on gynaecology and obstetrics.

'Maybe.'

The thought of a miscarriage is horrendous. It clarifies my desires. I want this baby.

Kate bought a pizza in Sainsbury's. Cheese and tomato again.

Worked till 3 am.

Tuesday 5 November

I am working on my film script again, even though I'm not being paid. I had promised myself that I wouldn't do any more unpaid work. But the film is my only realistic possibility of making a substantial amount of money before the baby arrives. Unfortunately none of my wealthy producers is willing to pay a rewrite fee. So I am gambling on the film's success, hoping that it'll provide food and clothes for my baby and self-respect for me.

I've admitted to Kate that I have a slight preference for a girl. She is sticking to the approved line: she doesn't mind if it's a boy or a girl, as long as it's healthy.

Whenever I've visited friends who have little boys, it's always like visiting a war zone.

I went swimming this afternoon at Dulwich Baths. After half an hour, the shallow end was cordoned off for a children's swimming class. In the hall, parents sat waiting, doing crosswords, staring into space, trying to tame their toddlers. When you're pregnant, people say you're 'in the club'. If Dulwich Baths is a typical example of the membership, I'm not sure this is a club I want to belong to.

Parents look tired and miserable an awful lot of the time. Yet they all say, 'Having kids is the best thing I've ever done.' When they describe their wonderful life in more detail, they talk about sleeplessness and pooh and fighting and tantrums.

Then they say they wouldn't have missed it for the world. I can't help wondering, do I want to miss the world for this?

At work today, Kate went to the toilet twice within an hour. Her colleague Debbie said, 'Is there a reason you've been to the toilet twice?'

'No.'

A minute later, Kate told Debbie that she is pregnant.

'I knew it! I knew it!' said Debbie, and gave her a hug.

Kate has been imagining that Debbie has been looking at her. Debbie admits that she has.

Through our kitchen window we could see the fireworks on Peckham Rye.

'We're having a baby!' Kate reminded me for the umpteenth time.

'I know. I am happy about it,' I said. 'It's just that at the moment I can't feel all the benefits but I'm very aware of the inconveniences. Haven't you got any qualms?'

'I have in the long term. In the short term, I'm looking forward to having six months off work.'

A friend emails me with news that a mutual acquaintance has become a father. 'The labour was very quick – so much so that Nick delivered the baby by himself in the living room.' This is even more impressive when you know that Nick only has one arm.

Worked till 4 am.

Wednesday 6 November
In the wee hours of the night, in the depths of sleep, I heard Kate shout, 'Ow!'

I woke up abruptly and saw that she was out of bed. 'What's up?'

'I just stubbed my toe on the stool.'

Panic over.

Parenthood begins before your child is born. You live with a dread of something going wrong.

So much for keeping it a secret. When Kate came home from work, she said, 'I told three people today.' One of them had guessed.

Thursday 7 November
Email from Ava. The last time I heard from her, a couple of weeks ago, she was ecstatic about being pregnant. Today she writes: 'Another thing, Andy – I'm no longer pregnant. I lost my baby, which was very sad.' That's all she says about it.

It reminds me how fragile everything is.

At the National Portrait Gallery, I wandered around an exhibition of photographs taken by young people from Peckham. They had taken photos of people in their lives whom they regard as heroes. There were several photographs of mothers, but only one of a father. All the mothers were praised for their loving natures and for 'teaching me about responsibility'. The comment about the father was: 'He can fix cars. He can sometimes repair videos that have been stood on.'

Kate went to bed straight after supper, saying, 'I've never had such bad headaches in my life.' I gave her a shoulder and back massage and was told to press gently.

Friday 8 November
We sleep like spoons. I wrap one arm around her, resting my hand on her belly. It feels as if I'm holding both of them. It feels as if there are three of us in the bed.

Kate got up for work. After breakfast, she got back into bed to snooze for an extra half-hour.

When she got home this evening she said, 'I'm absolutely exhausted.'

Saturday 9 November

Kate slept through most of the afternoon. Later, we were walking through the station at London Bridge.

'I don't know why I'm so tired.'

'It's because you're pregnant,' I reminded her helpfully.

'But I've slept a lot.'

'You just have to do what you feel like doing.'

She feels like lying down.

For supper we went to Sarah and Micky's house in Tufnell Park. Sarah asked how we liked our flat. I said, 'We like it, but it feels a bit small sometimes, and it's about to get smaller.'

'Why?' asked Sarah.

'Because soon there are going to be three of us living there.'

They seemed pleased for us. Sarah said, 'But Andrew, you said that you'd never have kids.'

I said, 'I didn't. I said I might never have kids.'

Micky said, 'It's a male defence mechanism. But it gets you in the end.'

It certainly got him. They have three kids now, aged 11, 9 and 6.

Watching Sarah being a mum and Micky being a dad over many years helps me feel confident that it is possible to cope. On the other hand, it's less reassuring to hear that all their friends with kids are separating and divorcing. Sarah suggested optimistically that, by having kids in our mid-30s rather than our mid-20s, we might avoid all that. We'll see.

As we left, Sarah said, 'I can't imagine Andrew as a parent.'

I was a bit offended by this. I reminded her that she has let me babysit her kids in the past.

She said, 'No, it's just that I can't imagine you giving up all your free time, and I mean a hundred per cent of it.'

Sunday 10 November   Week 13

This is the beginning of the second trimester.

Kate dreams about it more than I do. Last night she had a dream that we went for the first ultrasound scan and saw the baby and it talked to us. It turned out to be the nurses playing a joke.

We'd intended not to tell anybody about the baby until after the first scan, which is next Thursday. But good friends of ours are visiting London.

We decided to tell them when we met for lunch. Just before pudding, I said quietly, 'By the way, we're having a baby.'

Sophie hadn't heard. 'What?'

'We're having a baby.'

Clare hadn't heard. 'What?'

'We're having a baby.'

By the time I'd said it three times, the whole table had heard. These are some of our best friends. Of all the people we've told, they seem most pleased for us.

Dan asked me when it's due.

'The 25th of May,' I told him. 'About one o'clock in the afternoon.'

'What, really? Can they say what time it'll be?'

Dan is a 30-year-old single man whose friends don't have kids, so he doesn't know much about it. I used to be as ignorant as he is. Now I know words like *cephalic* and *meconium*.

It's interesting to see the different ways that friends react to the news.

Some childless friends respond by reassessing their own situation, as if our pregnancy is a challenge to their own lifestyle. It seemed to make Dan reflective and despondent. He asked me how long Kate and I have been together. I said, 'We've been going out for three and a half years and living together for one and a half years.'

Dan said, 'I'm just thinking what I've been doing for the past three and a half years.'

He has an enviable life: a job he likes, plenty of friends, time to travel. I was surprised by his regretful tone. Perhaps he is feeling the first inklings of dissatisfaction with the array of amusements that fill our lives. This feeling was one of the things that made me more open to the idea of having children.

When people with kids hear that you're about to have kids as well, their pleasure isn't entirely selfless. Our pregnancy is seen as an endorsement of their own life choices; and they're delighted that you're about to become as trapped and miserable as they are.

Over the years I've had many arguments with Sophie about Christianity. She admitted recently that her opinions have changed and she no longer calls herself a Christian. She told me this reluctantly, knowing that I would regard it as a victory. Now, as a mother of two, she looks upon my imminent fatherhood as a victory for her. She said to me, 'Andy, I have to say that I find it personally satisfying.' There was no way I could stop her feeling a bit smug.

Sophie said to me, 'It's all worth it.'

Her husband, Jack, said to me later, 'It's worth it ten times over.'

They are generous people and they have offered us an atticful of baby equipment.

A friend of a friend of a friend was having a birthday party, so we all went there, even the dog. I didn't know anybody, but there was champagne and cake, so I was quite content. One of the guests was a young woman with Down's syndrome. She leant against her father's shoulder. It reminded me that the scan on Thursday will indicate the likelihood of our baby having Down's syndrome. If there is a high probability of Down's, we will have the option of an abortion. Seeing this friendly and vivacious young woman at the party has made me dread that choice even more. I don't like what the situation is revealing about my own feelings about disability. I just hope that, on Thursday, it's only good news.

I am happy. I realised this in bed tonight, and it wasn't only because I'd just had sex.

Monday 11 November

I should be grateful that we're having sex at all. I read this today:

> Having a baby dramatically affects women's sex lives, a survey has found. On average, couples have sex half as frequently during pregnancy as they did before. This drops even further after the baby has been born. The survey of 500 women for *Prima Baby* magazine found couples made love 10 times per month prior to the pregnancy, five times a month during and four times a month after the baby is born. Two thirds said they were too tired or stressed for sex after the birth of their baby. Many said sex was the 'last thing on their minds'.

As I was reading this on BBC News Online, my new mobile was lying on my desk next to my computer. I have joined the 21st century. Until now I've lived quite contentedly without a mobile phone, but I've got one now so that I can be contacted in case of baby emergencies.

When a text message arrived, the text on my computer screen started to shake violently. If the mobile can do that to a computer, what is it doing to my head?

Tuesday 12 November
Despite feeling nauseous, Kate hasn't vomited during the first three months.

This evening, she came to me for a hug. 'I'm worried.'

'What about?'

'I can't feel anything. And I haven't been sick.'

'That's normal at this stage. In the second trimester you stop feeling so tired and sick.'

'What if it's dead?'

'It's not dead. And we'll see it on Thursday.'

'I'm worried about that as well. What if it has Down's syndrome?'

'The chances of that are very small. There's no point worrying about it. Our baby is perfectly healthy.'

'You don't know that.'

Wednesday 13 November
Feeling excited about the scan tomorrow. Looking forward to seeing our baby for the first time. I've been feeling optimistic about what we're going to see. Kate is worried. She wants proof that it is alive. I tell her that the chances are high that everything is perfectly normal. But now she's got me worried.

Kate is planning to eat a custard tart before the scan because she has read that sweet things make the baby move around. (A couple of weeks ago she read that bitter things make the baby move around. The more I read, the less I know.)

Thursday 14 November
We arrived at King's College Hospital at the appointed time and waited 50 minutes to be called. It was a typical London waiting room, full of people of all shapes and shades, faiths and fashions. Fifteen other pregnant women were there ahead of us, most of them with a male partner in attendance, a few with female companions and some on their own. The women wore lipstick and the men wore shirts; everyone had made an effort.

One man was reading a book called *How to Make Money from Property*. He had splashes of paint on his shoes. He reminded me of Peter, the husband in *Emma's Diary*; in the most recent photo, Peter is sitting in his kitchen with a pot of paint and brushes, renovating the house like a real man, setting a good example for the rest of us.

The woman doing the scan, Sandra, was chatty and cheerful. She squeezed cold gel on Kate's abdomen, just above her pubic hairs. I've been talking to the baby through Kate's belly button but the baby is much lower down than that.

Our baby appeared quite clearly on the monitor. 'Look, it's moving!' I said, as excited as a child on a trip to the aquarium. We hadn't expected it to be so active. Its little legs were kicking wildly and it kept turning round. Maybe Kate overdid it with the custard tart.

We saw the baby's body in profile, its beating heart, the two hemispheres of its brain. Everything looked normal.

Sandra said that she could assess the risk of Down's syndrome if we wanted her to. She said some parents don't bother because they're certain they'll have the baby regardless of that.

We said that we would like to know the risk.

Sandra took measurements and the computer produced an estimate of the statistical probability of Down's syndrome. A 33-year-old woman has a 1 in 368 chance of having a baby with Down's syndrome. Using the measurements, the computer provides a more accurate calculation of the risk; in our case the chances of the baby having Down's syndrome are 1 in 1,257. We can be absolutely certain by putting a needle through Kate's stomach and taking a sample of the fluid around the baby, but this has a one per cent chance of miscarriage.

'But it's your choice,' said Sandra, 'it's your pregnancy.' She did not use the word amniocentesis. Although she was obliged to offer us the option, she described it with a subtle brutality that was probably intended to put us off the idea. There was no need. We had made up our minds already. We said no thank you.

We no longer have to think of our baby in terms of food. All the books say the baby is the size of a strawberry, a chocolate-chip cookie, a cob of corn. Now we know the baby is 6.7 centimetres from rump to crown.

Afterwards I felt relaxed and happy. If I hadn't gone to the loo for a pee, I wouldn't have noticed that my hand was shaking.

Sandra kept several images of the scan for the hospital's records and gave us two to take home and show to everyone we meet. At reception, we were given a report of the scan and charged £2 for the two photos. In one image the baby is face up, in the other face down.

It's definitely not dead. As we walked away from the hospital, jubilant, Kate said to me, 'It was waving, did you see?'

Kate works around the corner from the hospital. We went there to make photocopies of our baby. We popped into the office of one of her colleagues, Eric, who knows she is pregnant. He has photos of his kids on the wall and was excited for us. 'It's 6.7 centimetres long,' said Kate. Eric tried his best to look fascinated.

Eric says that seeing his kids on a scan had a massive effect on him. Until then he'd just thought 'She's pregnant' but after the scan he realised 'We're having a baby!'

Kate's delight was all over her face for the rest of the day. 'There's a baby in there!' she said tonight as if she hadn't really believed it until now.

After weeks of fearing the baby was dead because she couldn't feel anything, tonight Kate thought she could feel the baby moving inside her (even though you're not supposed to be able to feel anything until weeks 18–22).

I have a photocopy of our baby on my desk.

A happy day.

Friday 15 November
'I'll miss having the baby inside me after it's been born,' said Kate.

'You say that now. Wait five more months and you'll be desperate to get it out of there.'

My film producer phoned with bad news. Ivan of Matador Pictures, who had promised to provide £5,000 for the writing of the next draft, is now saying that he won't give us any money at all until he sees more evidence that the project is guaranteed to go ahead. I said, 'Ivan is a cunt.' Ollie said, 'I know, but we can't tell him that. He's giving us 40 per cent of our budget.'

Clare, Nina and Dan came round for dinner. They brought us a bag of presents to celebrate the news: Nutella, anchovies and dill cucumbers in anticipation of Kate's strange food cravings (there haven't been any so far, unless you count a fondness for cheese and tomato pizzas); a large candle for romantic evenings alone while we still have the chance; and a giant pair of knickers (size 22) for Kate to grow into.

Kate showed them the images from the scan. They made appreciative noises without being as impressed as we are. They found it hard to discern the baby's body amidst the blobs of black, blurs of grey and splotches of white. Dan said it was like looking at constellations of stars and being told that there's a plough in there.

'Look, there's its head,' I said impatiently. They still couldn't see it. It's easier for us to interpret because we saw the scan. For other people it's like one of those Magic Eye pictures where you have to relax and defocus and wait for the image to appear.

Saturday 16 November
In a shop in Dulwich Village, Kate bought some maternity trousers. I told her that they look nice.

She stayed up late, till half past nine.

Sunday 17 November   Week 14
We bumped into a friend on Lordship Lane. When we told her that we're having a baby, she said all the right things without seeming hugely excited. I am a bit disappointed with people's reactions. How dare they react as I used to react? I realise now that many times over the years I've been insufficiently ecstatic when friends have told me about their pregnancies.

But you never know if the news has special significance to other people. Perhaps they want a baby? Or are wondering if they should want one? Perhaps they've suffered miscarriages? The news of our pregnancy might have unwelcome associations for some people, so we can't be offended by their lack of rapture.

The bookshop in Dulwich Village had 10 per cent off all books today. And a free glass of champagne when you walked into the shop. Kate had to watch me drinking champagne. She borrowed my glass and wet her lips, just for a taste. It's a lot easier being the expectant father.

I found a book called *Misconceptions*, Naomi Wolf's account of *Truth, Lies and the Unexpected Journey to Motherhood*. I bought it with Kate's encouragement but I'm not sure it was a good idea. Throughout the evening Kate kept exclaiming in horror and reading out passages. One woman says that feeling the baby move inside you is like 'having a sackful of ferrets in your stomach'.

Monday 18 November
Met two friends for lunch in Soho. Told them about the baby. They asked the usual questions. Am I pleased? Was it planned? Are we going to get married? Yes. Yes. No. I felt awkward talking about it with Rob. Last year he and his partner, Beth, were seriously injured while travelling

in Peru. Somebody had hidden smuggled gelignite under Rob and Beth's seat on the bus and it blew up. Beth died of her injuries.

Today, as we parted at the Embankment, Rob said 'congratulations' with a touch of irony because it's such a cliché. But it was generous of him to say it. When your own life has been devastated, you can end up resenting other people's good fortune.

Nor was I looking forward to telling Ava, who is visiting from New Zealand, when I saw her tonight. I considered not mentioning the pregnancy because of her recent miscarriage, but that seemed like a dishonest and short-term solution. I could have told her by email, which would've given her time to absorb the information before responding. But I decided that it would be better to tell her in person. Now I'm not so sure. She seemed momentarily shocked by the news. We discussed practical issues such as maternity pay without mentioning the emotions of the situation.

Kate joined us for supper in The Chelsea Kitchen. Afterwards, we said goodbye to Ava at the tube station. The last thing she said was, 'Let me know how it's going for you.'

On the way home, Kate asked me if I'd told Ava about the pregnancy, because Ava hadn't said 'congratulations' or anything to acknowledge that Kate was pregnant. Obviously the subject is too painful. Maybe I should have kept my mouth shut.

Kate has been feeling more nauseous than ever before. When we were in bed, as I tried to kiss her goodnight, she turned away, repelled by my breath. Which isn't that bad.

Tuesday 19 November
We went to King's College Hospital for the booking-in appointment.

When you go to a real hospital, you quickly realise that it's not like the hospitals on the television dramas. The staff aren't all nice-looking, dedicated and efficient. The receptionist was chewing gum and didn't know which form to give us.

The maternity wing is a brand new building. The rooms are clean, bright white and yellow. But the computers don't work. The midwife taking Kate's details had to write everything down on a piece of paper. Again Kate's name had been written down incorrectly. It doesn't inspire total confidence in their procedures.

Kate was told that she'll have another scan at 23 weeks. Then she'll attend the hospital once a month until 36 weeks. Then she'll go along every two weeks. She was told what foods to avoid, including pre-prepared salads. She was given forms to apply for a parent education workshop and a breastfeeding workshop. She was offered another form for free prescriptions and dental care. Four vials of her blood were taken to test for rubella, syphilis, hepatitis B/C and HIV.

Then we had to fill in a long form about Kate's medical history. She was asked about her history of sexually transmitted diseases and the regularity of her periods. She was asked about her family's health and if there were any abnormal births in her family. I wasn't asked anything. The members of staff hardly looked at me. To make myself feel useful I held all the forms and booklets.

Kate was given four categories to describe her relationship status: married, separated, single supported or divorced. The peculiar term 'single supported' didn't appeal to us, so in the end she chose 'other'.

Finally we were asked if we had any questions. Kate wanted to know how many births result in a Caesarean section. The midwife said about 25 per cent, but she didn't know how many of these were elected Caesareans. There is a general belief that doctors are too eager these days to resort to Caesareans because it makes life easier for them. The midwife tried to reassure us that the doctors in this hospital aren't like that. She said, 'They're not sharpening their scalpels.'

This phrase stayed with me for the rest of the afternoon.

The midwife also said that if a woman has been on the labour ward for a long time, the doctors might become impatient with her lack of progress and be tempted to intervene to help things along. Her advice was to delay coming into the hospital too early in the labour.

I can't see that happening. When Kate goes into labour, we're not going to dawdle at home. When are we supposed to begin the journey to the hospital, when the baby's head is sticking out?

Kate asked about home birth. The midwife said that about 8 per cent of pregnant women choose to give birth at home. 'The hospital beds are hard, and the floor is hard.'

But Kate has decided that she doesn't want to give birth at home. 'I think I'll feel more relaxed in hospital.'

Sophie has put us off home births. She chose a home birth the first time she was pregnant. After the baby was delivered, she started to haemorrhage on the carpet and had to be rushed to hospital in an ambulance.

A quiet evening at home. Suddenly Kate shouted out, 'Why does it have to be so painful?' She was reading Naomi Wolf's book. She read out a section that reports that American doctors in the 19th century believed that women giving birth endured more agonising pain than any Civil War soldier injured on the battlefield.

Wednesday 20 November

As we emerged from a cinema on Shaftesbury Avenue, I told my friend Louise about the baby. She gave me a peck on the cheek and a hug. Then she said, 'Oh no, you're going to become really boring.'

Meanwhile Kate was at work telling her bosses that she will be requiring maternity leave. She has only been in this job for a few months. Her general boss received the news with equanimity. But her immediate boss was resentful. The first thing she said wasn't *congratulations* or even *when is it due?* She said, 'Was it planned?' As if the pregnancy was a conspiracy against her.

Thursday 21 November

There's so much to do. Sanding the floor, painting and grouting the walls, finding and erecting a towel rail we both like (so far that search has occupied 15 months), finding and installing a light – and that's just the bathroom. Repairing the light switch and attaching a smoke alarm in the bedroom, fitting a dimmer switch in the kitchen, getting the boiler serviced, stripping and varnishing my desk. Kate also wants the window frames preserved, the chimney stacks repointed, extra shelves for pots and books, a new table for the TV. And then we want to move house.

In bed tonight, with the lights out, I felt my first flash of fear at the thought of the unending responsibility that lies ahead. A little person is going to need me. I'm afraid of failing him/her, and afraid that I'm going to lose important things from my life.

According to Roddy Doyle, I'm being a typical man by thinking like this. Talking on Radio 4 today about the genesis of his novel *Paddy Clarke Ha Ha Ha*, he said, 'I had my first child. Like most men, confronted with the birth of a child, I started thinking about myself.'

Friday 22 November

Kate talks to the baby. On a tube journey that was particularly noisy and smelly, she reassured the baby that everything was OK.

Hired a car. Drove to Yorkshire through fog and rain. Arrived at the B&B before midnight.

As we got out of the car, she said grumpily: 'You've left the lights on.'

'All right!'

I turned the headlights off, not easy when you're carrying seven bags.

In the long history of marital squabbles, this wasn't quite on the scale of Richard Burton and Elizabeth Taylor in *Who's Afraid of Virginia Woolf?* But for us it felt like a significant dispute. In bed Kate quoted a line she'd just read in the Naomi Wolf book about pregnant women: 'Everybody needs a pal.' So I promised not to be irritable for the next 18 years.

Who's my fucking pal?

Saturday 23 November

In bed I put my arm around Kate. She said, 'Don't press on my bladder.' Her bladder seems to occupy her entire body. Touch her anywhere and she wants to urinate.

In the morning we went to visit Kate's granny, Harriet, in Glen Rosa, a Methodist rest home for elderly people. She is 90 years old. There are 33 residents in the main house and another 14 in the separate annex for people suffering from dementia. Out of 47 residents, only 1 of them is a man. (The prospects for me aren't good.)

We haven't told her granny about the baby yet. We're waiting until tomorrow when Kate's brother Phil will be here with his wife Chloe.

Kate told her French grandmother, Mamie, on the phone last week. Mamie raised Kate's mum on her own. A few years ago Mamie advised Kate never to become a mother. 'Don't have any kids,' she said. 'They stop you living your life.' But when Kate revealed that she is pregnant, Mamie was delighted. Kate's mum was in the room with Mamie at the time. When Mamie, 89 years old, put the phone down she stood with her hands on her hips and she kept saying, '*Ça, c'est des nouvelles! Ça, c'est des nouvelles!*' (What news! What news!)

This afternoon we went to Dawn and Colin's wedding. Dawn's father had a seven-page wedding speech, but it was a good one. He reminisced about walking along Offa's Dyke with his daughter. It began to rain and Dawn, whose rainproof jacket had recently been washed, began to foam.

Later in the bar he told a few of us, 'I do implore you, if you have kids, do something with them. I can't remember her school years, they just went.'

Sunday 24 November   **Week 15**
We went to visit Harriet in the rest home.

Phil and Chloe were there with their daughter Holly. Chloe is pregnant again. She and Phil told Granny that she'll be getting 'another grandchild'.

This seemed like a good opportunity, so Kate said, 'Well actually Granny you're getting two extra grandchildren.' Granny's smile suggested that she was pleased. The strength of her feeling couldn't be contained and after a while she said: 'Well, well.'

Harriet is full of stories. But this is a good one. The use of ultrasound scans to examine the foetus in the womb was pioneered by Kate's aunty's dad. His name was Ian Donald and he was the Professor of Midwifery at Glasgow University. He had a patient whose husband worked at the nuclear power plant near the city. Out of curiosity, Ian Donald accepted an invitation to visit the power plant. There he saw the huge nuclear boilers whose internal walls had to be examined regularly for cracks. When Ian heard that ultrasound waves were used to detect flaws, it gave him an idea. He wondered if ultrasound waves could be used to examine the inside of the womb, which was a mystery to doctors. Helped by his knowledge of radar from his wartime experience in the RAF, he did tests using lumps of beef. Eventually, ultrasound scans for pregnant women were the result.

Ian Donald was a passionate anti-abortionist. He would be horrified if he knew how his invention is being used in some parts of the world. In India, some people pay for an ultrasound scan specifically to detect if the baby will be a girl. A female foetus is often aborted in a culture where the parents of a bride are traditionally obliged to pay a dowry. The cost of the ultrasound scan is regarded as a financial investment. The advertisements say: 'Better to pay 500 rupees now than 50,000 rupees later.' Even though female foeticide is now illegal in India, it has been estimated that 10 million female foetuses may have been terminated in the past 20 years.

Chloe advised me to do all the things I won't be able to do when we have a baby. 'Read books, newspapers. Go to the cinema. Go on holiday. Going on holiday is no longer a pleasure when you have children. Going on holiday used to be my favourite thing in the world. Now I dread it. The stress.'

Kate and I drove along the M62 to Warrington to visit my parents. I told my mum that I had an early Christmas present for her and handed her a small parcel. She removed the wrapping paper and found a rectangular picture frame containing the image from the baby's scan. Mum was as pleased as I'd expected. Soon she was texting the news to everyone she knew, even people in New Zealand. She offered to come to London to babysit for us, a round trip of 440 miles.

My aunt and uncle, Gillian and Bernard, came to visit. More hugs and kisses. They reminded us how childbirth has changed over the years. My uncle wasn't present at the birth of his children. He was watching cricket when he was told that he had a daughter.

Monday 25 November

I went to see my dentist in Warrington for a check-up. He told me that his 20-month-old baby wakes him and his wife at four o'clock every morning. 'But it's wonderful seeing the world through the eyes of a child … and it keeps you young.' As I was leaving, his final words of wisdom were: 'Go to the cinema now.'

Another day, another granny. We went to visit my nana in her flat on a council estate in Orford. She is 88, mentally sharp but physically frail. I showed her the two images from the scan. She looked and said, 'What is it?'

I said, 'It's a picture of your next great-grandchild.'

She was chuffed. 'I'm so pleased. And I'm pleased for your mum as well.'

This was a significant admission. Nana and my mum don't always get along. When my mum became pregnant in the 1960s, she wasn't married, so Nana threw her out of the house. After I was born, my mum and I were welcomed back. But relations between my mum and her family have remained uneasy through the decades.

Things said 40 years ago haven't been forgotten. One day, when I was a baby, my mum was in town with her Aunty Agnes and me. They saw people they knew. As they approached, Aunty Agnes told my mum not to admit that I belonged to her. 'Don't say it's yours. Say it's Oliver's.' Oliver was my mum's married brother. Even in the 1960s, according to my mum, the attitudes in the family were very Victorian. 'Nobody went to Aunty Win's funeral because she had run away with a married man.'

In the last ten years, births outside marriage have risen from 30 to 40 per cent. That's nationally, not just within my family.

Not so long ago, my baby would've been a cause of shame for my family. Now they're pleased for me. I'm pleased that they're pleased.

My Aunty Joan turned up, the youngest of Nana's six children. When I told her about the baby, she couldn't speak for a moment. 'I'm choked,' she said. She and Nana looked at the scan pictures. After a while Joan said, 'Which way up is it?'

We drove back to London. In bed, Kate read some more of that bloody Naomi Wolf book. Reading the chapter about Wolf's traumatic experience of giving birth, culminating in an enforced Caesarean, didn't help Kate go to sleep. She turned to me and said: 'I'm scared.'

Tuesday 26 November

We have decided to heed people's advice and go on holiday while we can. We've booked train tickets. We're going to Paris for four days in December.

Kate's conversational skills are deteriorating. 'I've been feeling queasy and farty,' she said when she got home from work. 'I've done two huge poohs today.'

Later, we were sitting on the sofa. 'Look at that!' she said, drawing my attention to her cleavage.

It's like waving a £20 note in a beggar's face. No, a £50 note.

Wednesday 27 November

Email from Nicola in Paris. She says her baby sleeps from 9 pm until 8 am. It gives me hope.

Kate nearly died tonight. She stayed out late with friends from work. A colleague, Eric, gave her a lift home. On the road from Wimbledon they were nearly in a crash. An oncoming car turned right, across their path. Eric braked and was forced to swerve across the carriageway. Luckily no other vehicles were coming in the opposite direction at that moment. Shortly afterwards, Kate felt a twinge in her tummy. When she got home she needed a hug.

Kate says that she gets out of breath just by walking a short distance.

She says: 'I think I'm at the stage where people might look at my stomach and think I'm pregnant but not say anything in case I'm just fat.'

These people are wise to keep their mouths shut. I once tried to make friendly conversation with a woman who was cutting my hair. I looked at her in the mirror and said, 'When's it due?'

But she wasn't pregnant. She was just a bit chubby.

'*What?*' she said. She was merciful, and didn't stab me with the scissors or give me a diabolical haircut. I gave her a big tip and never went back there again.

Thursday 28 November

This morning we went to see a solicitor on Lordship Lane to prepare a will. We are leaving all our possessions to each other. If we both die at the same time, everything will go to our children. We also have to nominate a legal guardian to look after our children if we are both dead. This is tricky. It's a lot to ask. And it makes you assess people in unkind ways. Kate suggested two of our friends, but I wouldn't feel comfortable about letting them bring up my kids. They're nice enough people, but I wouldn't want to inflict their neuroses and bad habits on my children.

Kate came home from work in a cuddly mood. We went to bed but one thing didn't lead to another. We are both frustrated. She is sorry that she doesn't want sex. I am sorry that I do.

So we lay there, thwarted. A bubbling cauldron of feelings. And they call this 'settling down'.

She tells me that her libido will come back, but I'm not so sure. Last night I read a mother's complaint in the Naomi Wolf book: 'I wish someone had told me what having a baby can do to your sex life.'

Sophocles lost his libido around the age of 70. He said, 'I am very glad to have escaped from this, like a slave who has escaped from a mad and cruel master.'

So, only 33 more years to go.

Friday 29 November

Our fridge was full of food but nothing that Kate wanted. She fancied something 'raw'.

'Such as?'

'Corn on the cob ... cheese and tomato pizza ... and one of those chocolate puddings. Oh, and bran for my constipation.'

I don't see what's raw about a chocolate pudding. I made an emergency trip to Sainsbury's. It makes me feel as though I'm contributing.

I think it was my dad who taught me the importance of contributing. He never did.

My mum and stepfather have been clearing out their attic. I have salvaged bags of old letters, scripts, notebooks. Tonight I was sorting through two decades of verbiage when I came across a page of scrawled notes about my dad. They were things I wrote down when my mum started talking about him one day about ten years ago. I'd forgotten a lot of the details until I read them today.

His name was Bruno Brunasso Cassinino. He had green eyes. He was good-looking. He came from Turin. He spoke four languages. He worked as 'a posh waiter' in a hotel. She met him when she was on holiday in the Isle of Man. He visited her in Warrington. She went back to the Isle of Man the following year to work. She bumped into him. I was conceived.

She worked at a pub in Finchley, North London, for four months before she had to admit to herself that she was pregnant. Back in Warrington, she went to see Dr Taylor. She panicked. She told him, 'I've got sinus trouble.' He gave her something for it. Next day she went back and told him the truth.

Nana ranted and told my mum to leave the house.

Mum stayed with her brother Oliver and his wife Judy for a couple of days.

Then she stayed with Aunty Agnes. Agnes said she couldn't let my mum stay there after I was born because Mum had no man.

So my mum went to stay with friends near Blackpool.

(It wasn't until years later that Mum told me the 'friends' were nuns who ran a hostel for unmarried mothers. 'One person helped me to keep sane during all of this and that was a nun. Sister Monica.' Years later, Mum took her some flowers and a box of chocolates. Sister Monica said, 'Nobody's done that for me before.' My mum told her, 'Nobody did for me what you did.')

I was born on 3 June 1965. I had a cleft lip and palate and I was taken to another hospital where I was kept in an incubator. The girl in the bed next to my mum said, 'You had a baby?' My mum said, 'Yes, he's here.' She rocked the empty cot next to her bed. She could 'hear' me making noises. The girl screamed for the ward sister and Mum was taken away. She was in shock.

When Nana first came to see me in hospital, I looked past my mum and smiled at Nana with my one bottom tooth showing. Nana said, 'He's trying to get his feet under the table.' It worked. Nana told Mum to come home to Warrington.

Mum got a job but made the journey every day to see me in Alder Hey Hospital on Merseyside. Often the buses were cancelled and Mum had to walk all the way back to Warrington in the freezing fog.

After six months in hospital and several operations to repair the cleft lip and palate, I was allowed home.

We lived with Nana and my mum's younger sisters and brothers in Margaret Street in a terraced house with an outside toilet, no hot water and no bath. By this time Nana's husband, who was often drunk and violent, had left and not come back.

Mum sent a letter to Bruno. He wrote back saying that he had been 'infatuated' but not in love. They had no further contact. She says she doesn't hate him now and wouldn't object if I went in search of him.

I was in my late 20s when she told me these things. I was 35 when I eventually made the trip to Italy to look for my father.

Reading these scrawled notes now makes me even more determined to be a positive presence for my child and for Kate. He was the worst kind of parent and my mother was the best kind. I know which I'd rather be.

Saturday 30 November

In the afternoon Kate looked distressed. 'I'm fat!' 'You're not fat, you're pregnant.' We have this conversation at least once a day.

We met Tony at a Japanese restaurant, Wagamama. I told him about the baby. He is squeamish and was keen not to be shown the images of the scan. He raised the topic himself, saying with an apprehensive tone: 'You haven't got one of those pictures, have you?'

He just wanted to chat about the football results and his new girlfriend. I can't help feeling slightly disappointed by the reaction of some friends who seem to be too self-involved to talk about me.

It's happening already, the realignment of friendships. What does the average baby cost, not in terms of money, but friends? It will require a conscious effort to maintain contact with friends like Tony who are members of the 'anti-natal classes'.

Sunday 1 December   Week 16

The 312 bus took us slowly from Peckham Rye through London's hinterland to Addiscombe, a suburb of Croydon. We saw Denise and Claude's new house and their new baby, four-week-old Thierry. He spent the whole afternoon sleeping. He was no trouble at all. It gives me hope.

Denise and Claude didn't read any of the pregnancy books but everything seems to have worked out well. It is possible to give birth without Miriam Stoppard. During the pregnancy Denise suffered from dehydration, gestational diabetes and bleeding, which makes us realise how lucky we've been so far.

Tales from the battlefront. Denise tried to describe the pain of giving birth 'because it's better to know what it's going to be like'.

'When you push,' she said, 'it's like being cut in two. Nothing prepares you for the pain.' I've never heard Denise swear, but she admits to saying 'Jesus Christ!' during the 25 hours of labour. She said, 'But it was helpful having Claude there with me.'

Claude didn't seem convinced about his helpfulness. 'I looked at her and I knew that she was alone.'

Kate asked what it was like for him.

He said, 'Horrible. Horrible. I will never forget it. You feel so useless. You want to do everything, but you can do nothing. I saw the way she looked at the baby the first time. It was not good. It was as if she was thinking: *bastard.*'

And now?

'Every day is like Christmas Day. He is a gift.'

Denise intended to breastfeed Thierry but he was reluctant to cooperate. The nurses provided a bottle, so Denise ended up bottle-feeding him. The first time Claude fed his baby, he gave him too much milk and made him vomit. 'Now I don't watch television while I'm feeding.'

Claude says that, like all parents, he and Denise will make mistakes. But he doesn't feel less capable than the millions of ordinary people who muddle along and manage to raise children.

Kate has said that she enjoys the feeling of kinship with other pregnant women. There is consolation in knowing that other people are in the same boat; or, if not in the same boat, at least adrift in the same sea. So I felt sorry for her tonight. She went to an antenatal yoga class and she was the only person there apart from the teacher.

Monday 2 December

I read the first chapter of Rachel Cusk's book *A Life's Work*. 'My mother has always been fairly honest about her own experiences of birth. When the time comes, she says, take any drugs they offer you.'

I also peeked into *Emma's Diary* to see what she and Peter are doing in week 16. They are painting the nursery yellow. That's one job we don't have to worry about. We haven't got a nursery. Our flat is so small that we're not sure where we can fit a cot in our bedroom. Things will work out, that's what I keep telling myself. I remind myself that my gran raised six kids in a cramped terraced house. This is true. It's also true that she didn't enjoy it.

Kate is almost at the end of the Naomi Wolf book. She is reading about severely depressed mothers stuck at home while their husbands are out at work. She said to me seriously, 'You won't leave me on my own, will you?' I promised her that we will cope together. No matter how unhappy we become, at least we will be miserable together.

Kate told her Uncle Harry about the baby. He said, 'What are you doing that for?' He is a father of two.

According to the books, the second trimester is a time of renewed energy and well-being. It hasn't happened yet. Kate goes to bed after the ten o'clock news and I stay up late working or reading or wasting time.

Tuesday 3 December

Now and then this kind of thought comes into my mind: What if Kate was in an accident and the baby died? What if Kate dies in childbirth? What if there's something wrong with the baby? What will happen to them if I die? I keep these fears to myself. If Kate mentions that she has had a similar daymare, I tell her not to be silly, not to worry, everything's fine. But I am just as bad, equally prone to morbid thinking. The world is more alarming. We have more to lose.

Today I read this: 'On average parents lose between 400 and 750 hours of sleep during the first year.'

I went to the Bloomsbury Theatre to see various comedians, including Jeremy Hardy, Mark Thomas and Michael Moore. John came along and I told him the news. He is my oldest friend and I was wondering how he'd respond.

It's hard to say 'Kate is pregnant' or 'We're having a baby' without sounding like a character from a bad soap opera, so I resorted to my usual ploy of just handing over the image from the scan.

He stared at it for a few seconds and then said: 'Kate?'

I nodded. Who else would it be?

'Brilliant,' he said, and shook my hand. After a moment, he added, 'You'd better start making some fucking money, mate.' After another moment, he said, 'I wondered if you were trying but I thought it was rude to ask.' After another moment, he said, 'This is the problem, I have no big life events.' As if this news is about him. Our pregnancy seems to prompt other people to reassess their own lives.

My oldest friend's response couldn't be described as an outburst of emotion. There are reasons for this. We are men. We are English. We are middle class. (As one of the comedians said tonight: 'I hate being middle class. The money's good, but apart from that …') We just aren't like that. I wouldn't want him to burst into tears and give me a kiss on both cheeks. But it's pitiable that we are conditioned to deprecate and minimise one of life's most significant events.

This is why having a baby puts your friendships under strain. It's not just that caring for a child leaves less time for other people. The insufficiency of our friends' excitement emphasises their detachment. Their reaction to our situation draws attention to our separateness and distance from other people, even those closest to us. Pregnancy exposes the limitations of friendship.

'Only connect,' wrote E M Forster. Our most intense experience of connectedness, of mutuality, of other-centredness, comes from the process of having a child. I suppose that's one good reason to have kids.

My mum has given us £150 for Christmas. It's a lot of money and it's not as if they're rich. I phoned to thank her and she said, 'Well, you'll be needing it.'

Wednesday 4 December
After attending a talk about birthing pools last night, Kate thinks she might elect to have a water birth. The contractions are supposed to be less painful in the water. Apparently there's no danger of the baby drowning. A baby only starts breathing when it encounters air that is a different temperature from its body. The hospital provides a sieve if the woman craps in the water. It'll be my job to scoop the poop.

I spent half an hour in W H Smith this afternoon, browsing through this month's pregnancy magazines. According to them, our baby is 5 or 6 inches long now. This is quite big. I mentioned it to Kate later. A mistake. Now she is worried that she isn't as large as she should be. 'What if it's stopped growing?' I had to get the tape measure to prove that her waist has expanded by 4 centimetres in the past 2½ weeks.

'I want it to move!' she said. It is moving. We saw that on the scan, but she won't be able to feel it for another month or so.

We are living by a new calendar. Holidays are no longer identified by seasons but by trimesters. The pregnancy books urge people to go on holiday during the second trimester, which is allegedly a hiatus of well-being between the nausea of the first trimester and the grumpy immobility of the third. It is recommended as a final opportunity for togetherness before the baby enters your lives 'like a hand grenade' (as one mother describes it).

So we've decided to go to Italy in March. We don't really know how Kate will feel by then, but Italy doesn't require a long flight; it has decent medical services in case something nasty happens; and Rome gives us the choice of frenzied sightseeing or lazing in cafés.

Thursday 5 December

Worked until 4 am last night. The baby is one deadline I can't ignore.

The disheartening thing is that I'm working with film producers who are millionaires, and they're expecting me to work for nothing. Ivan, who has reneged on his promise to pay me £5,000 to rewrite the script, drives a £95,000 Mercedes and his family owns acres of property in the South of France. He told Ollie, 'My father would be disappointed in me.' 'Why, because you're working in the film business?' 'No, because I'm working at all.'

Kate was told at work today that she is entitled to full pay for eight weeks, then half pay for ten weeks plus statutory maternity benefit. So our baby won't starve. Not all babies in the world are that lucky.

Her belly was aching tonight. I assured her, with my authoritative knowledge of obstetrics, that this is perfectly normal. Her skin, her muscles and her organs are being stretched and squashed. She is entitled to ache.

Friday 6 December

'The baby is growing fast,' I read today. 'The body grows bigger so that the head and body are more in proportion.' That's a relief. On the first scan, the baby looked like an alien. Luckily I'd seen images from scans, so I knew what to expect. When scans were first introduced, many parents must've thought, *What the hell is that?*

This week our baby is the same length as a banana.

The last episode in this series of *Friends* concluded with Rachel giving birth to a daughter, the first baby in history to be born without an umbilical cord. This scene reduced Kate to floods of red-faced tears. She asked for a hug. The tears were for our baby, not Rachel's. 'What if something's wrong with it?'

I told her that 99.9 per cent of babies are born perfectly healthy and normal. We both knew this was an exaggeration, but she stopped crying and returned to her plate of cauliflower cheese.

At one o'clock in the morning, Kate was woken by the noise from the flat downstairs. Jonathan was in another one of his rages. Usually we can hear Jane shouting back, but this time we couldn't hear her at all. I phoned their number but nobody answered. Kate didn't want me to go downstairs. I phoned again and let the phone ring for a couple of minutes. Still no answer, but all was quiet after that.

Saturday 7 December

Kate says she is more frightened and nervous about things in general. That's why she didn't want me to go downstairs last night to tell our neighbour to stop shouting at his wife. She thought he might stab me. I said, 'But what if he was attacking her?'

'I'd rather she died than you.'

We went to an Indian restaurant on Shaftesbury Avenue to celebrate Louise's birthday. Louise asked to see a picture of the scan, which I happened to be carrying in my pocket, so I showed her. Our baby was exhibited on the table among the wine bottles and party-poppers. The idea of birth and parenthood provoked an outbreak of revulsion among some of the women in their 20s.

Louise was unimpressed by the scan photo: 'I thought you said you could tell it was a baby?' Disappointed by my friend's ignorance, I pointed out the baby's head and body. For some reason, nobody could see it. Some of them seemed unwilling to look too closely, as if it were something contagious.

The afternoon has made us aware of our separation from the tribe of childless people.

During supper we watched the end of a film called *Sliding Doors*. This is supposed to be a romantic comedy, but if you're a pregnant woman it's a tragedy about a woman whose boyfriend is unfaithful to her.

In bed, Kate was tearful and inconsolable about the prospect of my infidelity. She told me, 'It isn't just me now. You'd be being unfaithful to the baby as well.' This is unfair. I have promised her that I'll never be unfaithful. And I'm not exactly overwhelmed with opportunities anyway. Most days the only women I meet are the cashiers in Sainsbury's where romance is unlikely to blossom: bored 16-year-old girls and 60-year-old men with beards aren't my type.

She says that she is feeling more vulnerable and emotional. In the past few days she has been reduced to tears by a sitcom and a romcom. These things should carry health warnings: Not Suitable For Pregnant Women.

Sunday 8 December   **Week** 17

Kate was walking strangely. She was bent over. 'I've got bad stomach cramps. I can't stand up straight.' I gave her a gentle stomach massage, subject to careful instructions. 'Don't press too hard, you'll squash the baby … here … put your hands on the skin and just move it around.' It seemed to do some good.

John came to visit us in the afternoon and told us about his mate Pete who is separating from his wife. Since the birth of their second child five years ago, they have had sex twice.

At the moment I am remarkably unconcerned about the lack of sex. Occasionally when we embrace the familiar feelings spread through me, but I think of other things and the sensation passes.

Three friends came round for supper. Kate told them that she is pregnant. They laughed at the number of pregnancy books on our shelves. But they all ended up sitting round the table reading them, fascinated and horrified by the photos of women giving birth.

Men are imbeciles, according to the pregnancy magazines. Every article aimed at men talks to us as if we're emotionally and intellectually retarded. One of the magazines advises me to talk to my baby after it is born – 'even though you might feel silly having a one-way conversation'. In fact, I began talking to my baby weeks ago, even before it had ears.

But I'm wrong. We do need to be told, apparently. One of our friends is a speech therapist who says that some parents don't talk to their children at all. When the child is 18 months old and still wordless, the parents complain to doctors and speech therapists that their child isn't speaking.

Kate mentioned that she has been reduced to tears by sentimental television programmes. Carla said, 'It's begun already. Your brain has started to die. You're becoming cow-like.'

Pregnancy and birth are a continual source of amusement for friends who aren't about to undergo it. Kate mentioned that she might choose to have the baby in the birthing pool at the hospital. John said, 'Does it have lanes? Fast labour, medium labour, slow labour?'

Monday 9 December

For parents, the future is a foreign country; we will do things differently there. In ways we can't imagine, our lives are going to be different when the baby is here. So we have to make practical decisions about the unknowable, such as whether or not we need to get a car. The average baby seems to travel with more luggage than Queen Victoria. Some of the pregnancy magazines recommend cars bigger than our living room.

We are obliged to make a sensible decision on behalf of the people we are going to become. This involves relinquishing, to some degree, the people that we are. The only car I've ever owned was an MG Midget. It was essentially an oversized go-kart, a roller skate with a 1,500-cc engine. Every journey was an adventure; I never knew if I would arrive at my destination before something fell off or exploded. Now we are test-driving character-less Fords and reliable Renaults.

But I expect that future journeys will retain an element of uncertainty and danger. We'll never know for sure if our child is going to explode. Even an old MG whose gearstick had a habit of coming off in my hand seems a sedate alternative to the average toddler.

Kate was in bed by half past nine. 'I'm very tired. Don't know why.'

I washed up, tidied the kitchen and carried on working.

Tuesday 10 December

Worked until 5.30 am last night. So I wasn't awake when Kate got out of bed and discovered that the boiler wasn't working. It was 2 degrees outdoors and 2 degrees indoors. It's an old boiler. A replacement would cost £1,300.

When I eventually surfaced from my coma around 1 pm, I found a note from Kate informing me that a heating engineer would be visiting during the afternoon. Eventually two men turned up. Real men. Men who know how to mend things. It turned out that the boiler had merely overheated; it had cooled down during the day so all the men had to do was reignite the pilot light. For this they charged £76.38.

A couple of weeks ago there was a letter in the *Daily Telegraph*: 'I've always thought one should, if possible, have three children: one a doctor, one a lawyer and one a plumber.' I recommend having a fourth child who is a heating engineer.

Kate stayed up until 11 pm. 'I'm fat!'

'You're not fat, you're pregnant.'

Every night we examine her bump. When she lies on her back, her stomach slopes gently upwards like the South Downs. Tonight we noticed a steeper hillock starting around her navel, more like one of the foothills in the Pyrenees.

There's always the unspoken anxiety that something might go wrong. Every day that passes is a relief.

Wednesday 11 December

The most enthusiastic reactions come from friends who have kids of their own. This evening on the phone I told Eddie, father of two daughters. He sounded genuinely pleased. 'That's really excellent news, man.'

Eddie is a child of the 60s and a big fan of Bob Dylan. But I've known him for 20 years and I've never heard him say 'man' before.

Last week Kate phoned the woman who organises the local National Childbirth Trust antenatal classes. We have to go along on four Thursdays and two Saturdays. The cost is £120.

Now leaflets have arrived from the NCT, including a sample of their newsletter. One article promises 'childbirth without fear' using yoga and hypnotherapy. Oh yeah? Who are they kidding? I've heard different things about the NCT. One father told me that it gave him 'a sense of belonging'. Another friend warned me that 'the NCT is a cult'.

As part of her clinical skills training as a psychologist, Kate is doing a Family Therapy course. Today she had to compose a kind of family tree called a genogram. Symbols are used to represent family members and their relationships. Women are circles. Men are squares. Pregnancies are triangles. Miscarriages are triangles with a cross over them. Instead of using a triangle, Kate decided to represent our unborn baby with a star. Apart from the scan, it was our baby's first public appearance, the first time its individuality has been recognised and recorded. She brought the genogram home. An untidy array of simple shapes, like a child's drawing, it is a kind of inverted Christmas tree with the star at the bottom. Looking at this family tree was the first time we've seen the baby in the context of the complex matrix of people to whom it's related. And we saw our new role. We are no longer an end but a means. Now we are not just dangling branches. We are roots.

We were sitting quietly together and she announced, 'I haven't poohed for two days.' I get regular updates, whether I want them or not.

Thursday 12 December

Last night, in the dark, waiting for sleep, I felt a sudden chill of trepidation at the thought of the responsibility of it all.

Kate says we need to put our baby on the waiting list for a place in the day nursery at work. This is subsidised by her employer, the NHS, but the prices are still frightening. For a child aged three months to two years, a place in the nursery for one day per week costs £27 (£1,377 per year). For three days per week, the cost is £81 (£4,131 per year). That's more money than I've earned in some years. As a playwright, I'm used to working for low pay or no pay. Now my job is more likely to cost me money than make me money. Time has suddenly become very expensive. It makes me think about all the time I've squandered throughout my adult life. It was worth millions.

The main advantage of money is that it stops you having to think about money. It allows you to get on with other things. Until now I've tended to agree with Epicurus who wrote that 'the possession of the greatest riches does not resolve the agitation of the soul nor give birth to remarkable joy'. Now I will have to rethink my attitude to money. I will have to earn some.

Today on the phone Ollie surprised me by saying that they've found another investor and in principle the film is once again 100 per cent financed. I've heard this before. I've learnt not to get too excited. This is merely a rumour of a hint of a possibility of a glimpse of a faint light at the end of the tunnel. But that's good enough for me. Hope is restored. I felt something ease inside me. I've been suffocating for the past few weeks. The pressure is a physical sensation. You only realise its strength when, just for a moment, it eases its grip.

THE DIARY

Friday 13 December

Kate isn't usually a grumbler. 'I want to sit down!' she whined in the book-shop at Waterloo Station. On the train she flopped into a seat. 'I've gone all weak and tired suddenly.' I had failed in my duties. Although I was carrying most of her luggage, I had forgotten to bring along a supply of food for emergencies like this. I still haven't got used to taking responsibility for someone else's appetites.

We are in Paris. At the Gare du Nord an American women inserted her American Express card incorrectly into the cash machine. It was stuck. It took five different nationalities to find a pair of tweezers to extract her card. I was in holiday mood so I found the incident amusing, but Kate was impatient.

'You're so fucking grumpy,' I told her.

As I said it, I could sense Miriam Stoppard frowning at me. She says on page six: 'There's no greater help to a pregnant woman than an interested and sympathetic partner.'

We are staying with Kate's mum, Susanne, who has rented an apartment near Bastille while she is working in Paris for a month. After an evening stroll along the banks of the Seine, we ended up on Boulevard St Germain des Prés where we paused to rest in a café called Les Deux Magots. This is where Picasso, Verlaines, Giacometti, Rimbaud, Mallermé, Sartre and Simone de Beauvoir used to come. They probably all shared a coffee. It took me a moment to translate the prices into the new currency. I worked out that a *chocolat chaud* costs five nappies.

I'm going to try to stop worrying about money. I am starting to bore myself.

I showed Kate's mum the images from the scan. She couldn't see the baby. But it's so obvious to us.

Saturday 14 December

Saturday night in Paris. What to do? Obviously you spend an hour and a half choosing maternity clothes in a shop called Natalys.

It is cruel to be in Paris and forbidden to drink wine. Deciding that the benefit to the mother was far greater than the risk to the baby, Kate allowed herself a small glass. We are becoming more relaxed about the rules, which change with each person/book/country you come across.

We found a little restaurant in the Place du Marché, off the beaten track.

We entered, wondering what variety of local characters ate there. At the next table there were eight people from Birmingham.

It's hard for our baby to be a non-smoker. We asked the waitress if there was a non-smoking area but she said, '*C'est Paris. À Paris c'est perdu d'avance.*' (It's Paris. You are lost before you start.)

Soon there were people smoking at every table. Even one of the waiters was smoking. You'd think it was illegal not to smoke. In fact, in small restaurants like this where separate areas for smoking aren't available, the entire restaurant is supposed to be non-smoking.

A large proportion of miscarriages and cot deaths are linked to smoking and passive smoking. Miriam Stoppard tells me that the chemicals absorbed from cigarette smoke limit foetal growth by reducing the number of cells produced in the baby's body and brain. Nicotine makes blood vessels constrict and therefore reduces the blood supply to the placenta, interfering with the nourishment of the body. The babies of mothers who smoke are on average 200 grams (7 ounces) lighter than those of mothers who don't smoke, and low birthweight babies can have health problems and are less likely to survive. The incidence of premature births almost doubles in smokers. Smokers are more likely to have children with various types of congenital malformations, especially cleft palate, cleft lip and abnormalities of the central nervous system. Smokers have nearly twice the risk of miscarriages and stillbirths.

Sunday 15 December   **Week 18**

We went to Pigalle to visit Nicola, her partner Thierry and their baby Marc, who was born four months ago. Nicola told me that Marc is impeccably behaved. He sleeps all night and rarely cries. I held him for five seconds and he began to cry.

Their fourth-floor apartment is small and damp, yet they seem to be coping. They have 24 books on pregnancy. Nicola said that, after a while, she got sick of reading pregnancy books and returned to novels. I am feeling close to that stage of development.

Oh to be in April now that Paris is here. Undaunted by the drizzle, we strolled around the local streets with Marc strapped to his mum's chest in what the French call a *kangourou*.

Back at the apartment we watched, fascinated, as Nicola gave Marc a bath. Even babies aren't spared the French obsession with toiletries. Nicola extracted a sterilised swab from a plastic wrapper and wiped it across Marc's eyelid. She used another swab for the other eye. After this, a small plastic capsule of saline solution was squirted up each nostril. Nicola said, 'He doesn't like this.' I'm not surprised.

She rinses his bottles in mineral water.

Now that he is here, Marc's parents aren't taking any chances. There were complications during the pregnancy. Nicola had an amniocentesis as she was told that her chances of having a baby with an abnormality were comparatively high. 'Imagine sixty marbles in a bowl,' her doctor told her. 'You have to pick one of them, and only one of them is abnormal.'

Marc was born healthy after a Caesarean.

Monday 16 December
Today we were eating lunch (OK, cakes) in a café in the Marais when the barman began to smoke. We were sitting at the bar next to a NO SMOK-ING sign, so Kate complained. He said that the sign referred to the area beyond where we were sitting. I said, '*Ma femme est enceinte*,' (My wife is pregnant) and he extinguished his cigarette.

Some of the French lingerie adverts are unsettling for a man who hasn't had sex for five weeks. And it's not just the adverts for lingerie. Shoes, cars, washing powder, anything.

At the entrance to the Métro station at Bastille, there was a classic scene: a youngish man and a youngish woman were clinging to each other in a passionate embrace, inert except for the rhythmic chomping of their mouths. When I looked back, they were still going. When I turned around for a final time, just as Kate told me to stop staring, they hadn't moved. Oblivious with lust, they were a reminder of past times. While most of the pleasures of parenthood have yet to appear, the old excitements are still prominent in my mind.

We went to see the Matisse–Picasso exhibition at the Grand Palais. Some of the people were more eye-catching than the paintings. There is some truth in the old joke. Monogamy leaves a lot to be desired.

According to a survey, 25 per cent of pregnant women are afraid that their male partners will be unfaithful during the pregnancy. A different study found that adulterous women were more likely to be unfaithful during the days when they were ovulating. It's foolish to deny the power of biology, or to be a victim of it. When you love someone, you don't stop noticing other people. This is what commitment means. Brave people aren't fearless; if they feel no fear, their actions require no courage. In the same way, committed people aren't lustless.

Kate is more sensitive to smells these days. Some of the Métro platforms stank of sewage and urine. When we took the evening train back to London, we moved seats because some kids were eating crisps and the smell was making Kate feel sick. We moved to the other end of the carriage where things weren't much better. Someone was eating a McDonald's and the whole carriage had to share the McOdour.

We're still looking for names. Kate bought a French magazine called *Parents*. As she browsed through its pages, she said to me, 'Theo is a nice name.'

I said, 'Theo means God. It seems a bit immodest.'

An article in *Parents* argued that New Man isn't much better than the old man. New dads spend 14 minutes per day cooking, compared to mums' average of 69 minutes. Dads spend 11 minutes doing housework and 2 minutes washing clothes, whereas mums devote 28 minutes every day to these tasks.

Tuesday 17 December

Kate had two dreams last night. In the first one, after giving birth, she went for a long walk around London, leaving me sleeping with the baby. When she eventually returned, everyone was disapproving of her absence. In the second dream, I delivered the baby and the nurses took it away. When they brought it back, it was much bigger. Later we discovered that it wasn't the same baby, even though the nurses said this was impossible.

Kate asked me, 'Have you had any baby dreams?'

'No.'

'It's not fair. It's a roller coaster.'

Her pregnant friend had a dream about giving birth to a hamster. Then she lost the hamster somewhere in the house. Then she accidentally sat on it and killed it.

Another appointment at the hospital. The woman we saw last time had said that we might be able to hear the baby's heartbeat during this visit. We've been looking forward to this. But first we had to sit in the waiting room for two hours. If you're having your baby in an NHS hospital, the first rule is: always carry a book.

After we'd been sitting there for an hour and a half, they started playing classical music. Kate phoned work to cancel some meetings. After half an hour of Vivaldi, her name was called. This time our midwife was called Annabel. That's a nice name for a girl, I thought. An hour later, I had gone off the idea. Now I wouldn't call my dog Annabel.

She started off pleasantly enough. She asked how the baby was. She asked how Kate was. She even asked how Daddy was.

Annabel explained that there are always delays because there are enough midwives available but not enough rooms. This seems strange, since the maternity department is situated in a brand new multi-million pound building, which only opened a few weeks ago.

Annabel asked if we've booked our NHS antenatal classes; we said that we have, but we haven't received confirmation of our booking yet. She said that we wouldn't hear from them until week 34. The classes begin in week 35.

Kate said that she would need more than a week's advance notice so that she knows which days to keep free in her diary.

Annabel said that 'pregnant women are forgetful' so it would be pointless to arrange the dates a long time in advance.

This doesn't seem to be the philosophy of the NCT, which has already given us the dates of their classes.

Annabel asked us when our baby is due. We said 25 May. She told us that if Kate hasn't given birth two weeks after that date, labour will be induced. She said this sternly as if she was expecting us to argue.

Then Annabel couldn't find our file so she disappeared for ten minutes. When she came back, she told us that today's appointment was completely unnecessary. As if it had been our idea. She said that we don't need to attend the hospital so frequently at this stage. This contradicted what we'd been told by the previous midwife.

When we tried to arrange our next appointment, Annabel suggested a Tuesday or a Wednesday.

Kate looked at her diary and asked if another day was possible.

Annabel said, 'Yes, how about … Tuesday?'

'How about Monday?'

'Can't you make Tuesday?'

Eventually Kate conceded defeat and agreed to come on a Tuesday.

Annabel looked at Kate and said, 'You look anxious.'

When Annabel left the room to get something else she'd forgotten – the results of Kate's blood tests – Kate turned to me and said: 'She keeps you waiting for two hours and then says that you didn't need to come at all! And then they project it onto you by saying you're anxious! Fuck off!'

There are three things tested at these meetings: 1) Blood pressure. Remarkably, Kate's hadn't gone up. 2) Urine. This is because 5 per cent of pregnant women experience diabetes as a result of the baby's hormones suppressing the level of insulin. 3) And finally we get to listen to the baby.

At this stage it is too early for Kate to feel it moving. Annabel warned us that our baby is only the size of a tennis ball and, if it was resting at the back of the pelvis, we might not be able to hear its heartbeat. She applied gel to Kate's abdomen and pressed a listening device deep into her belly button. We could hear Kate's breakfast, but not the baby. Annabel chased the baby around the pelvic region, like a destroyer hunting for a submarine. Kate's insides sounded like the depths of the Atlantic. 'Ow!' said Kate when Annabel pressed too hard. We were all starting to realise that our baby wasn't going to make an appearance today.

Annabel placed her hands on Kate's tummy and said, 'Can't you feel it moving? It is moving around a lot!'

Could this be true? Perhaps Annabel's experience made her especially sensitive to the baby's movements. I placed my hands on Kate's tummy and felt nothing. By now I had lost confidence in Annabel and I suspected that she was making it up.

Later we looked in the medical notes at Annabel's report of our meeting. Annabel had written one word: 'reassured'. This simply wasn't true. Her report should have said: 'pissed off'.

As always with large organisations, your experience depends on the individuals you encounter. Kate chose to come to the hospital for these antenatal appointments because she thought she'd get to know the midwife who might deliver our baby. Now we've been told that none of these midwives works on the delivery ward. This is disappointing, but in another way it is a relief. We're hoping that the midwives on the labour ward will be more efficient, and that the stupid ones are confined to these antenatal appointments.

Tonight Kate laughed scornfully at advice in one of the pregnancy books about being in labour. 'Don't forget to relax and enjoy it.' Kate groaned at the thought of what lies ahead. She threw back her head in anticipation of the agony, inadvertently mimicking the posture of the women in the photographs, none of whom seemed to be finding the experience relaxing or enjoyable.

I told Kate not to worry. I will be there (as the books recommend) with drinks, snacks, lip salve and coins for the phone.

Wednesday 18 December
People keep giving us advice. Some of it is rubbish.

My friend, a mother of two, has advised Kate to start rubbing her nipples with a rough cloth. This is supposed to toughen them up before the onslaught of breastfeeding. My friend found breastfeeding 'really painful'. It's like having a piece of skin sucked relentlessly, she said. Her husband is a GP and he came up with the cloth idea. (We were later told that this advice is completely wrong and that abrading the nipples with a rough cloth removes natural oils.)

'I feel bigger.' Kate thinks there was a growth spurt today.

She stayed up till midnight.

Thursday 19 December
I'm making an effort to have a social life while I still can, so I went to the monthly book group at Dulwich Library for a Christmas party. One woman was attending for the first time this year. She said it's difficult getting a babysitter in this area because there are so many kids. This part of South London is increasingly known as Nappy Valley.

One man is a journalist with two teenage children. He says that, if I want to work at home, I'll need earplugs.

A middle-aged woman said that she calls her pre-motherhood years BC. Before Children. And afterwards? 'It's overwhelming,' she said.

When I got home, Kate said, 'Come here, I want to show you something.'

I stood in front of her and she pushed her breasts together. She is still fascinated by her cleavage.

'Very impressive,' I said. 'Is that what you've been doing all evening?'

We've received a Christmas card addressed to Kate and Andy and bump.

The bump is suddenly bigger. It has the consistency of a large balloon. Or a Spacehopper.

In bed she said, 'I'm very happy.'

'So am I.'

It's true, we are. I'm not sure how that happened.

Friday 20 December

My financial situation has improved. At the supermarket checkout I dropped a £1 coin. It rolled away under the counter. I searched but couldn't find it. But I found a £2 coin instead.

A magazine article says that around week 18 '... you may be starting to feel remarkably sexy around now. Around a third of women say they do, and it's down to hormonal changes and an increase in blood and fluid in the entire pelvic area. But if you'd rather have a nice cup of tea, don't worry – another third of pregnant women go right off sex altogether.'

'Do you want anything?' I asked Kate after supper.

'Camomile tea,' she said.

I have been wondering if we'll ever have sex again. I am trying to be philosophical about it. I am wondering if I'll have to take up jogging again. Jogging got me through my adolescence.

Kate told me tonight that one of my duties when she's in labour will be to apply olive oil to her perineum.

This was news to me. I said, 'Olive oil?'

'It's natural.'

'Olive oil is natural. Rubbing it on your private parts isn't natural.'

But she has read somewhere that this helps the elasticity of the area, making tearing less likely during labour. I'm just going to do what I'm told. Tonight in bed we had a trial run with remarkable results.

We were trying to have sex but the early signs weren't promising. We were attempting a side-on position recommended for sex during pregnancy; this would have been feasible if my penis was 10 inches longer. Eventually we decided to change position. Kate suggested introducing the olive oil.

I felt foolish as I walked naked to the kitchen and returned with a small pool of olive oil in a bowl.

I said, 'This isn't going to work. It's extra virgin.'

I was wrong. I am pleased to report that sex is possible during pregnancy. It seems that the books are right when they say that the extra hormones in a pregnant woman's body may accelerate and intensify her arousal levels.

It was noisy sex. No doubt it says more about me than her, but she isn't usually one of those women who shout out during sex. But tonight she did. She shouted out, 'I need to pee!'

If you're hoping to sexually arouse a pregnant woman, you must show extra consideration to one particular part of her body; I am referring, of course, to her bladder.

Saturday 21 December

Woke up at 6.30 am to carry Kate's bag to the train station. She is going away for a week. She is flying to the South of France to spend Christmas with her granny and her mum. I've decided to stay in London. One thing I'm not going to have so much of in the future is time alone. This week is a Christmas present to myself. I need to do some work.

Received an email from a friend who is travelling in South America. I prepared myself to cope with a flood of envy. But as I read her accounts of meeting sexy travellers, climbing volcanoes and watching ocean waves crashing on a sunny beach, I was surprised by my lack of resentment. I am pleased to be doing what I'm doing. Peckham on a grey Saturday feels like a satisfying place to be. Having a baby seems a worthwhile thing to be doing.

Sunday 22 December   Week 19

Worked all night on the film. Got to bed at 7 am. Before going to sleep, I listened to the headlines on the radio. After years of bombings, rapes, murders, famines and wars, I'm not often shocked by something I hear on the news. But today I was sickened. According to a police study about domestic violence, men often become violent when their partner tries to end the relationship or *when their partner becomes pregnant*. 'Pregnancy is often a time when abuse begins or intensifies. Nearly one in three cases started during pregnancy.' It's hard to understand some people.

I haven't looked at *Emma's Diary* for a while. In week 19 she feels the baby move.

Kate phoned from France. She still hasn't felt any movements. I'm hoping it won't happen while she's away.

Monday 23 December

Friends ask me if I want to know what sex the baby is. No, I don't want to know. It feels a bit like X-raying your Christmas presents.

Pregnancy is a time of physical discomfort for both of us. Kate has decided that she is only going to drink bottled mineral water from now on.

'You'll have to carry it,' she tells me, laughing. A French pregnancy book has convinced her that water from the tap is endangering our baby's health. If you believe everything in the books, you end up like Howard Hughes, paranoid about the things you eat and drink, fearful about the way you live your life. After a while, the risks to health are less damaging than the constant mental strain of self-surveillance and self-denial; a pregnant woman can find herself restricting her diet and limiting her activities so much that she becomes her own jailer.

Tuesday 24 December

Kate phoned and burst into tears. 'I had a fright this morning. I was turning the taps on my granny's bath when I felt a strong electric shock along both of my arms. Like static electricity but stronger than that. It's the wiring in this old apartment. I was crying afterwards. I felt fine again until I just started talking about it.'

I said, 'Don't worry, lovey. I'm sure the baby wasn't harmed.' As if I know.

More Christmas cards have arrived. People seem less interested in the baby Jesus than in their own babies. Their messages are a glimpse of things we can look forward to. A friend in South Africa writes: 'Ben is very cute, can say rhinoceros, which we think is pretty brilliant. And this morning he drew all over himself with pen, put toast in the video machine and watered the couches using his watering can. Oh fun fun fun.'

I caught the tube to Tufnell Park. In previous times I might've paid more attention to all the attractive women, but today I was more interested in the knackered-looking woman with a small child. I was admiring her pushchair technique on the escalators.

Went to Sarah and Micky's house for Christmas Eve cake and drinks. Just me, 7 other people and their 14 children. Occasionally we would hear screaming or sobbing from another part of the house, and one of the adults would sigh and leave the room.

Sarah said, 'You need a car, Andrew.'

I said, 'Eighty per cent of the world's parents don't have a car but somehow manage to raise their children.'

'Not in South London,' she said.

Practical Parenting has a whole section devoted to cars.

Wednesday 25 December
Woke up early and read 'Hell's Kitchen', a chapter in Rachel Cusk's memoir about motherhood. 'At its worst moments parenthood does indeed resemble hell ... I often think that people wouldn't have children if they knew what it was like ... there is in truth no utterance that could express the magnitude of the change from woman or man to mother or father ...' Merry Christmas.

Several friends have told us that we'll be good parents. There are moments when I have my doubts. I like having time and space to myself and I'm worried that losing these things will make me a resentful and miserable dad.

I've decided that now is a good time to calm down. I've been working frantically, staying up until the early hours, too busy rushing through life to enjoy it.

Kate phoned from France. They are having pigeon for Christmas dinner. I'm glad I'm not there.

John came round in his new Mini and we drove to Raynes Park to spend Christmas Day with Terry and Ruth. Chicken and champagne. Jenga, Abalone and Scrabble. John and I stayed up till 3.30 am, building a Jenga tower 34-storeys high, even though we are both 37 years old.

Thursday 26 December
Kate phoned from France. She can feel her stomach moving: it's not the fluttering of a kicking baby, but a tugging sensation as her muscles are stretched. She thinks she has got bigger since she left London five days ago. 'I think I've had another growth spurt. *[yawn]* But I feel fine. *[yawn]* I slept well. *[yawn]* I'm tired. *[yawn]* Sorry, I can't stop yawning. *[yawn]*' It was only 7 o'clock in the evening.

Her sister-in-law, who is also pregnant and feeling intensely sick most of the day, has been told by a doctor that 'It's a sign of a healthy placenta, if you're feeling ill.' Now Kate is worried that there's something wrong with her placenta because she hasn't been feeling ill enough.

'Doctors will say anything to make a pregnant woman feel reassured,' I said, trying to make a pregnant woman feel reassured.

Friday 27 December
I phoned Kate. The main news from France is: 'I've got terrible wind.'

We discussed stretch marks. Kate saw a news report about a French maternity ward. It showed a woman having an ultrasound scan in the 23rd week of pregnancy. Apparently this woman's stretch marks were like zebra stripes, thick pinkish-white slashes across her body. After seeing this, Kate went out in the afternoon and bought a tub of cream that claims to prevent stretch marks.

'I know, it's ridiculous,' she said. 'But you kind of get pulled into it.'

According to the books, the extent of stretch marks depends on your skin type and all the creams are useless; the marks are caused by hormonal changes rather than by the stretching of the skin; if you want to know whether you're likely to suffer from stretch marks the books suggest that you look at your mother's body.

Some of the pregnancy magazines still recommend the creams. These are the same magazines that rely on advertising revenue from cosmetics companies.

One argument in favour of the creams is that they make women feel better. Some magazines urge women to regard creaming as valuable Me Time. I'm not against Me Time, but can't they think of anything better to do with it? They'd get more benefit from going for a walk. But nobody makes money from that.

I squandered half the day watching Christmas television and *The Great Escape* for the 30th time. I should have been working. When I'm watching television these days, I can feel the baby watching me disapprovingly and saying, 'Why are you wasting your time, Daddy?' I already feel that the child is witnessing my life and I must be on my best behaviour.

Saturday 28 December

Work can bring out your best or your worst. Slow progress, lack of money, prolonged confinement and the company of liars and fools; the film business isn't bringing out my good side.

I am trying to finish a script before Kate comes home tomorrow. When she phoned this evening, I was tense and tetchy. 'Time is running out,' I told her. I shouldn't have said this. It made her think that I'm not looking forward to seeing her. I shouldn't be making her cry. 'What's wrong, lovey?' I asked, although I knew. 'I don't know,' she said, 'I've been missing you so much.' I have given her the impression that I'm not missing her.

This is something I'm not very good at, talking to people when I'm in the middle of working. But this is going to happen all the time. Children want to play. Children need to be fed, cleaned, monitored. I am going to be responsible for a creature with no control over its emotions or its bowels. Am I going to snap at my child every time it needs my attention?

I don't want to be the kind of parent that's always saying 'In a minute!' 'Not now!' 'Later!' Kate deserves better than that as well. This is the danger. Making money suddenly becomes more important when you're having a baby; if you're not careful, you end up working so much that you're less available to your loved ones when they most need you.

She says that I don't need to meet her at the train station tomorrow because her bag isn't as heavy as she thought it would be. 'I'll come anyway,' I said. This was the right thing to say. But I still feel bad because I don't really want to go.

One of the books contains a pregnancy diary whose author concedes that 'My brain is suet and I can't remember anything … I keep forgetting where I am in the middle of sentences.'

Does pregnancy make women slightly stupid? This is a controversial topic. I only have anecdotal evidence. This evening Kate said that she was enjoying the novel she's reading.

'What's it called?' I asked

After a silence, she said, 'I don't know. It's blue. Do you want me to go and look?'

'No, don't worry. You'll probably forget your way back to the phone.'

Sunday 29 December   Week 20
I forgot to water the houseplants while Kate was away, even though she asked me specifically. Now they are desiccated and dying. I can't blame pregnancy for my own stupidity.

Kate's flight landed on time. I went to meet her at Liverpool Street. She looked lovely. She is lovely. Her return has cheered me up. Back in Peckham, she phoned her deaf granny in France to say that she'd arrived safely. 'ANDY MET ME AT THE TRAIN STATION,' she shouted, 'HE CARRIED MY BAGS HOME.' This earned me maximum Granny Points.

We went to bed and ate French chocolates. Then we tried to have sex. This used to be an easy, natural thing. At this stage of pregnancy, sex is as perplexing and erotic as trying to fit two bicycles into the boot of a car. Finding a position that makes sex comfortable and feasible takes time. An hour and a half, in this case, with sulking and tears of frustration along the way. Her belly is bigger and there are numerous body parts that are sensitive or delicate. 'What are you doing?' I asked at one point. It turned out that she was trying to achieve another position recommended in one of the pregnancy books. It was like a wrestling match. The actual sex was concluded very quickly. Having got that far, we wanted to get it over with before anything else went wrong. But it was worth all the effort.

Kate is 'a bit worried' because she still hasn't felt the baby moving. Tonight she thought that she could feel a bubbling sensation. I put my ear to her belly and listened to gurglings that were difficult to interpret. One of the books says that you can hear the baby's heartbeat more easily through the cardboard tube found inside toilet rolls. I haven't noticed any of the midwives using these, but I decided that it couldn't do any harm. I went to the loo and returned with my instrument. I still couldn't hear anything distinguishable from indigestion.

Around now our baby is beginning to grow hair, eyebrows and eyelashes. Lines are forming on its fingers, creating its own individual fingerprints. The hands can grip firmly. Teeth are starting to form in the jawbone. Nerves and muscles have developed sufficiently for the baby to stretch its limbs. It is about the same length as a corncob.

Monday 30 December

Last night I worked until 5.30 am. When I went to bed, Kate was awake and had been for two hours. Insomnia is common among pregnant women, according to the books, along with heartburn, varicose veins, piles, constipation, breathlessness, tummy ache, itchiness, cramp, incontinence, swollen ankles and feet, pins and needles, skin tags, rashes and spots, gestational diabetes, stretch marks and backache.

It's easier being the dad.

One of the books says: 'Insomnia: scent your bedroom with two or three drops of lavender oil.' Our bedroom reeks of it. It makes me cough and keeps me awake.

Kate came home from work and started crying. This time it wasn't my fault. She had spent an hour on the phone arguing with a member of her family. I had to dissuade myself from picking up the phone and giving him a bollocking. Another argument would do more harm than good. A television writer once gave me some wise advice about working with producers: 'Pick your fights.' That's also a good tip for getting along with family.

THE DIARY

Tuesday 31 December

We've been invited to spend New Year's Eve with friends in Worthing. On the train from Victoria, there was a woman in a wheelchair; she had to sit in the dark and dirty guard's van with the bicycles and bulky parcels. That's one reason why I hope my child isn't born with a disability; disabled people are treated so badly.

At midnight we stood on Worthing's pebbly beach, watching fireworks exploding above the pier in a black sky. We clinked our glasses against the bump.

Later in bed, Kate said that she was feeling 'vulnerable' and 'cut off' because I've been working so hard. I am working longer hours because of the baby, and she is feeling neglected. We have become clichés.

Today's lesson. If you're hoping to have sex with a pregnant woman in a strange house, make sure she knows where the bathroom is, otherwise you waste valuable time during the inevitable toilet break. Even your heavy breathing is likely to put uncomfortable pressure on her bladder.

Wednesday 1 January

Kate fell over this afternoon.

But that wasn't the first trauma of the day. In the morning we had an argument. It was one of those arguments about nothing and about everything. She asked me to do something and I said I'd do it in a minute when I'd finished my cup of tea. She didn't like the way I said this. We both took offence and sulked for a while. These are emotional times. She has the excuse that hormones are flooding her body. I have no excuse. I was just panicking, wondering how I'm going to be able to work when I'm sharing a small flat with her and the baby. I suddenly felt trapped in an oppressive relationship. This feeling lasted for about 15 seconds, then I recovered my senses. We talked things over and agreed that, whatever the difficulties ahead, 'we'll work something out'. Trusting our future to these unspecified grounds for optimism, we cheered up and decided to enjoy New Year's Day.

Wild, wet and windy in Sussex. Local football matches were called off due to flooding. A train was derailed by a landslide. Despite the monsoon, we decided to go for a walk on the South Downs. One of our friends had forgotten his waterproof trousers, so he wore a skirt made from a bin bag. Sometimes the clouds lifted to give us a clearer view of the sheets of rain being blown across the landscape into our faces. It was great. We ate sandwiches and chocolates on the edge of a wood. Weary, damp, happy, we were descending along a footpath on the side of a hill when Kate's boots slipped in the mud and she fell sideways, landing heavily.

She quickly stood up again as if it wasn't a big deal. 'It's all right falling over, isn't it?' she asked me. I assured her that it wouldn't harm the baby, but it was unlikely to do her much good. We were both surprisingly calm about it. We've read that a simple fall is unlikely to endanger the foetus.

Thursday 2 January

Imagine having sex while being punched in the stomach. That's what it feels like when your pregnant partner is on top of you. It's difficult to be swept away by passion when a medicine ball is being bounced on your tummy.

That's what I discovered this morning after being woken by the sex-crazed succubus who has taken over Kate's soul. Her moods are unpredictable. I don't know if she's going to have tears or a twinkle in her eye. All feelings seem to be heightened. Emotionally, it's a roller coaster; sexually, it feels more like bumper cars. This is an improvement on a few weeks ago when our sex life felt more like one of those fairground games where you have to throw a ring over a wooden cube and you can never quite manage it and you never win the prize.

It's not so difficult to detect her emotional and physical changes. As she moves around the house there are unsolicited announcements, clues to her state of mind and well-being. 'Tired.' 'I've got mad hair.' 'Oh God.' 'Don't want to go to work.' She emerges from the toilet after 15 minutes and says, 'Constipated.'

This evening we met Dan and went to Clapham Picture House to see a Stephen Frears film. All the cinema adverts seemed to be aimed at childless 20-somethings, promoting a lifestyle of glossy, youthful, unfettered hedonism. This approach to life was in full swing in most of the bars along Clapham High Street. I felt like an outsider in my own city. In the evening, our cities belong to the childless young. Parents and children, like old people and tramps, aren't welcome on the streets. This might seem a natural and inevitable division until you look at countries like Spain and Italy where children are welcomed in restaurants. In some European countries, an evening out is a convivial family occasion, a way of life for people of all ages rather than a marketed lifestyle for the young.

All this is just a convoluted way of saying I'm dreading being stuck at home every night for the next five years. I just want to be able to blame my feelings of entrapment on social injustice rather than personal immaturity.

Afterwards we went to a Thai restaurant called The Pepper Tree. There was a baby at one table. This gave me hope that we're not going to be completely housebound and that our social life won't be confined to parent and toddler groups.

Dan told us that his parents took him to India when he was three and his brother was a baby. He is extremely optimistic that we will still be able to go travelling when we have children. Of course, Dan hasn't got any. Everyone we know who has kids says the opposite.

Between our worst fears and our wildest fantasies lies the truth. I like to believe that, if we really want to do something, we will make the effort and do it. Travelling with children might be possible after all. I have decided to be an optimist, while I still have the chance.

An American poet, Don Marquis, wrote this: 'an optimist is a guy / that has never had / much experience'.

Friday 3 January

I keep forgetting to walk more slowly. As we walked from the train station to our friends' house in West Dulwich, Kate was feeling breathless. 'Can you slow down?' She had to ask me twice. I would be a lot grumpier than she is. Five couples at the dinner party. Everyone feels at liberty to touch her bulging tummy. She says she doesn't mind.

Our friends' house has vast, stylish, expensively decorated rooms. It was easy to tell who has children and who doesn't. Our friend Craig was showing us his luxurious cashmere sofa. Lydia, a mother of two young children, asked immediately: 'Is it washable?'

Inevitably (so it seems these days) the discussion turned to children and pregnancy. Lydia had an interesting tip. Apparently, a tea strainer is an ideal accessory when you're breastfeeding. You cut off the plastic handle and place the strainer over your nipples; this dries them out by allowing air to circulate around them.

Saturday 4 January

Kate is much more cautious about crossing the road these days. She won't cross unless a car is a mere speck in the distance. When we do decide to step into a road, she runs across to the other side. Lately she has started clutching her belly as she does it.

She is usually the most easy-going, sweet-natured person in the world, but she was grumbling all day. She almost told someone off for parking in a space reserved for disabled people because 'they didn't look disabled'. In a shopping centre she glared at seven teenagers who were smoking underneath a large NO SMOKING sign. She is a human smoke detector; she can detect cigarette smoke from half a mile away.

Her heightened sense of smell means that I have to be careful about what I eat. When I said that I might treat myself to a veggie pastie from Greggs the Bakers, she said that she wouldn't kiss me afterwards. (I bought one anyway and, in fact, she still kissed me.) In the bakery her face was contorted with disgust at all the foul smells. My face must've shown my dismay that she is continually disgruntled. She told me off. 'You mustn't make me feel that I'm being difficult,' she said, being difficult.

I'm hoping that this is a temporary irritability. I have been assuming that, as she is a nicer person than I am, she will be a nicer parent. I have been measuring the kind of parent I fear I could be (resentful, impatient, bored) against the kind of parent I'd like to be, and also against the kind of parent I think she'll be (loving, generous, understanding). But pregnancy is a physiological revolution and parenthood is a psychological revolution. Who knows what kind of people we'll turn into? As well as wondering what kind of person our child will be, I'm wondering what kind of people we'll be.

There isn't much wood in Colliers Wood; there is a bus garage, a Burger King and a large shopping centre. Shopping is a surreal experience. Kate wanted to buy a computer. I asked the salesman for a leaflet with all the prices; he told us to look on the website. In other words, we needed a computer in order to find out how much it costs to buy a computer.

We took a Peugeot 206 SW for a test drive. The rear door was too narrow; getting a baby out of a child-seat would break your back. When I asked how much the car costs, the salesman wanted to know if we intended to buy it there and then. He said, 'I don't want to work out all the figures if you're not going to buy it today.' In other words, he wanted us to agree to purchase it before he would tell us the price.

I need to learn not to regard every slight ailment as a symptom of something sinister and baby-threatening. I saw Kate wince. 'What's wrong?' I asked anxiously. She said, 'My hair was tickling my ear.'

Sunday 5 January   **Week** 21

A friend, Steve, phoned from Japan to congratulate us. He lives in a small apartment with his wife and baby. He teaches English and is also studying for an MA in Japanese. He says it's impossible to work with a baby in the apartment, so he has been studying in libraries and on park benches.

I suppose I should be encouraged and inspired by such initiative. When D H Lawrence lived in Italy, he used to lie down in the woods and write novels and short stories and plays and poetry; he was so still and quiet that deer used to come up to him. I'm not sure if I'll be able to employ this working method on Peckham Rye, where the climate isn't like Tuscany and the wild creatures are more likely to mug you than nuzzle you.

Steve was present at his daughter's birth in a Tokyo hospital. He says, 'I couldn't see much through my tears.' His wife doesn't even remember that he was there. 'Every time I tried to do something, she just swore at me.' The tradition in Japan is for the man to cut the umbilical cord. Steve didn't do this. 'I was crying so much that they didn't think it was a good idea. They didn't even offer it to me. I was crying more than the baby.'

Things haven't been easy since then. But Steve's final message was: 'I love it.'

Some people are already asking us if we're planning to have more than one child. What I feel, and what I say, is this: 'Let's get the first one out first.' Kate is less circumspect. She just says, 'Yes.'

My friend Sarah, who is also an only child, has said to me: 'You can't just have one, you know that?' Her fourth child is due to be born in July.

Monday 6 January

Our baby is galvanising people who don't often get in touch. A long-lost friend phoned to congratulate us. She has a three-year-old son. She says that she is feeling a lot happier now that her divorce is going through. Despite everything, she says that 'children are so fulfilling, the peaks are such a joy that the freedoms you lose don't matter, and you feel more a part of the world, and you're less selfish'.

Yesterday Kate met a friend who has a two-year-old daughter. The father wanted to call the little girl Christina, but the mother wanted to call her Rosemary. In the end, the name written on the birth certificate was Christina. Now the father calls her Christina, but the mother calls her Rosemary. I'm sure the child will survive this; I'm not so sure about the parents. This is a situation we hope to avoid.

Some couples discover that a baby turns them into enemies rather than allies. It would be arrogant to believe this can't happen to us. I don't suppose anyone embarks on parenthood expecting it to lead to acrimony and alimony, but that's what happens a lot of the time. So far we haven't had to work too hard at our relationship. Perhaps that's what children can do; they can make your life at home seem like work rather than leisure. We'll see.

Pregnancy is a leap of faith. Until we've experienced parenthood for ourselves, we just have to trust other people's opinions when they say that it's worth it.

Tuesday 7 January

Kate went into labour last night. I had forgotten to pack a bag to take to the hospital, so I ran around the house trying to gather towels and slippers and various elusive items. It was a horrible dream.

We had A Quiet Night In. We ate in front of the television, watching an exploitative and entertaining programme called *Wife Swap* about two couples who exchange partners for two weeks. It was a glimpse into the chaos of family life. One family seemed to have modelled itself on a fascist state; the other family lived in a perpetual state of anarchy. One father refused to let his son leave the house for two weeks because of a minor misdemeanour.

'What would you do in that situation?' I asked Kate. She asked me the same question. We're testing each other and ourselves, wondering if we're equipped to cope with the challenges ahead.

I don't want my children swearing excessively or watching too much television. But this means that I will have to stop swearing excessively and watching too much television.

Kate still can't feel the baby. Every night I put my ear to her tummy and listen. A friend, a mother of two, says that when you feel your baby kick for the first time, you realise that it has been kicking for ages but you failed to identify the sensation. Her babies announced their presence with a pleasant fluttering feeling. 'Like having a butterfly inside you.'

Wednesday 8 January

People at work are starting to notice her bump. She is pleased. 'Crikey! What's that?' said one of her colleagues this morning. She sees people glancing at her belly as she walks past.

Does pregnancy make women stupid? Further circumstantial evidence has turned up. We went to a café on Northcross Road. As we were leaving, she realised that she had lost her gloves. She went back to our table but couldn't find them. She asked the waiter if he'd seen a pair of orange gloves. No, he hadn't. As he was saying this, I noticed that her hat was perched quite high on her head. Her gloves were inside her hat.

More snow. Peckham looks like Vienna. Children were clambering over giant snowmen on Peckham Rye. Local kids challenged us to a snowball fight. Cars were skidding. Africans were taking pictures of themselves in the snow, as if they had never seen it before. We ambled around East Dulwich, enjoying the crunching sounds that snow makes underfoot, and doing a few shopping chores. It's not the kind of adventure that people write books about, but we were happy enough. Being with someone you love is the nicest thing in the world. (As long as they love you back.)

'The supreme happiness of life is the conviction of being loved for yourself, or, more correctly, being loved in spite of yourself,' wrote Victor Hugo.

The boiler is broken again.

Thursday 9 January

'I think I'm feeling things,' said Kate. 'Kind of bubbles. It feels like one big bubble inside me, moving around.'

She has been worried because some people have said that her bump isn't very big for someone in the 21st week. She says that she would like to have a bigger bump. I keep telling her to enjoy it now while it's not too heavy.

She is waking up in the night a lot. She isn't cycling because she doesn't feel safe on the bike any more. But she is walking a lot and feeling better for it. Apparently there's evidence that exercising during pregnancy can reduce the length of labour by a third. We want to believe this.

Psychologists have a policy of limited self-disclosure, which means they don't reveal much about themselves to their clients. Kate is finding this is impossible when you're pregnant. Today her 13-year-old client was full of questions. 'Are you pregnant?' 'Is it your first?' 'Where are you having it?' 'I was born at King's!' When a social worker turned up, the girl passed on all this information to him.

Friday 10 January
In W H Smith I glanced at the shelves of pregnancy magazines and, for the first time, I felt sick of the sight of them. Some of the novelty is wearing off and the baby isn't even here yet. Have I peaked too soon?

Most of the world's mothers get their knowledge about pregnancy and childcare not from books or magazines but from their older female relatives. My mum used to work in a maternity ward so I've been hoping to benefit from the wisdom of a lifetime's experience. Tonight on the phone her only significant insight was that, during the last three weeks of the pregnancy, Kate will walk like a duck.

Kate says she felt 'a sense of loss' at work today. Most of the time she enjoys her job and she is beginning to realise that she'll miss it when she's on maternity leave. It's the first time I've heard her express sadness about some of the changes ahead of us.

'I think I can feel something,' she said. I put my hand there. We asked the baby to kick harder. I still couldn't feel anything.

Kate made a noise something like this: 'Nurrrggghw.'

'What?'

'It's exciting and … it's going to happen.'

The happening is starting to seem more real.

Saturday 11 January
We went for a walk and saw the sunset behind the chimneys from Peckham Rye. It's not the Serengeti – you're more likely to see poodles than tigers – but we like it. Kate can't walk as far as she used to. We only managed half a circuit of the park.

For several weeks she has been fascinated by her expanding belly button. This evening she showed me that the base of her belly button is now visible. 'Isn't that amazing?' Well, no, not really. She says that the belly button on some pregnant women turns inside out. This is one wonder of pregnancy I'm finding it hard to get excited about.

Sunday 12 January   Week 22
'I'm feeling things.'

'What kind of things?'

'Same as last night. Like bubbles inside. It feels like I want to fart, and then there's a feeling of release.'

So the magical moment, the first physical manifestation of the baby's movements, feels like a fart.

I cooked pasta with mushrooms tonight, the first time I've cooked in a week. Most evenings Kate starts preparing a meal before I even think about it.

One of my New Year's resolutions is to become a better cook. When we decided to live together, Kate was concerned that she would end up doing most of the cooking. I promised her that we wouldn't allow that to happen. Then we allowed it to happen. She is a good cook. She has a genetic advantage; she is half French. She can take 20 minutes to cook something that would take me two days of planning and worrying. I recently made a recipe from a book called *The 30-Minute Vegetarian*. It took me two and a half hours.

I used to work as a chef in an Italian restaurant in San Francisco. It was called Giorgio's but the owner's name was Tony. You could tell how long people had worked in the kitchen by how many burns they had on their arms. This was one of the things that motivated me to find another job after eight days. The thrill of making someone's meatballs wasn't enough to risk mutilation. 'All labour has dignity,' said Martin Luther King Jr, but he never worked at Giorgio's.

I am a dull cliché – a man who can't cook. But I am going to improve. I've said this before and nothing has happened. I've bought recipe books and then never opened them. But this time I am going to make a real effort. I want to be able to feed my child proper food. And I don't want my child to learn bad cooking habits from me. I don't want him to grow up living on cereal and toast like his dad used to do.

Monday 13 January
I worked until 7 am. I got into bed and snuggled against Kate's warm body. A minute later the alarm clock detonated and she had to get up for work. All day she felt more bubbles inside the bump.

She has lots of dreams. The recurring themes seem to be: Will I bond with it? Will I love it enough? Will I cope?

Last night she gave birth in her dream. It was quite a quick labour. Afterwards she was breastfeeding … not the baby, but me. By the time I had finished, there was no milk left for the baby. Kate sees this as a sign that she is worried about not having enough love to share between the baby and me.

Kate asked me: 'Has my bum got any bigger?'

I said no.

My bum has got bigger. I used to use the first notch on my belt. Now I am on the second notch. One day last week I had to use the third notch. Pregnancy is making me fat. We're less active than we usually are. And there's more food around. I caught sight of myself in the mirror today before I could suck in my stomach. I look about 15 weeks pregnant.

Kate kindly said that I'm not fat. She said, 'Anyway, we all put on fat over winter to combat the cold.' This is true, but we live in South London with central heating. My stomach is suitable for a long Siberian winter.

We watched a Channel 4 documentary about young girls who are obsessed with their body image. We were revolted. The premature sexualisation of young children's behaviour amounts to child abuse. One nine-year-old wears high-heeled shoes to the playground because she likes to be 'sexy'. She went to children's parties wearing four different kinds of make-up. When she grows up, she wants to be 'an aromatherapist or a pole-dancer'. Apparently some shops sell padded bras for seven-year-olds.

'Let's not have a girl,' said Kate.

Tuesday 14 January

Worked on the script until 4 am. Emailed it to Mike Barker, the director. At lunchtime I arrived at his huge house near Islington to discuss it. His kitchen is bigger than my flat. We talked in a purpose-built, purple-walled shed at the bottom of his garden. A father of two, he used to work in a room on the third-floor of his house 'but the kids were too noisy'.

I am continually looking to see how other parents arrange their lives. Mostly, this induces panic. London can give you the impression that raising children is impossible without a nanny, a four-storey house with five bedrooms, daily yoga classes, a personal trainer, £2,000 of photographic equipment, a four-wheel-drive Land Rover and an eight-seat Toyota. I have to keep reminding myself that everyone, one way or another, seems to cope.

I phoned Warrington to wish my stepfather, Trevor, a happy birthday. On the card I wrote: 'Happy 60th birthday – a good age to become a grandad'. He has never had kids of his own. I was 14 when he married my mum, and

I have never called him my dad or regarded him as my dad. Calling him my child's grandad feels like a way of acknowledging our relationship and what he has done for me, without violating my sense of self, my sense of independence. He hasn't been in the best of health since he retired, so I hope this new role gives him a boost. On the telly a couple of days ago I heard a man in his 60s saying that his grandchildren had 'filled a gap'. If Trevor has a gap, I hope this helps to fill it.

Kate and I went to bed at 10 pm, the first time in a month that I've been in bed before midnight. Lately she hasn't been suffering so much from insomnia, but tonight she couldn't fall asleep. I gave her a sympathetic hug and then, cruelly, went to sleep. At 2 am she got up to open a window. 'Hot. Can't breathe.' After that I couldn't sleep either. I rubbed her back, which is starting to have aches and twinges.

Wednesday 15 January
She was about to walk up three flights of stairs in an office building today when the receptionist noticed that she was pregnant and escorted her to a lift which only people with a pass are allowed to use. This is the first time she has received special treatment because she's pregnant.

This evening I cooked pasta with a bean sauce while she sat at the kitchen table with a critical eye. She got annoyed because it was taking so long. The pasta would've boiled quicker, she said, if I'd put more water in the pan. She says, 'I'm not complaining, I'm just commenting.'

This whining is only remarkable if you're familiar with the serene, calm, cheerful person that she was before armadas of hormones started rampaging around her body.

'Constipated!' she cried out to the gods. Throughout the evening there was a litany of discomforts: 'Oh God! I just feel stiff and tense!' 'Can't breathe!' 'My stomach is so hard!' The evening concluded with a despairing realisation. 'Oh God! It's going to get worse!'

I said: 'Why are you surprised? You've read all the books about backache and … and about all the other symptoms.'

'I know, but I didn't think they'd apply to me.'

Similarly, I suspect that parenthood, despite all the books and the classes and the role models, is still likely to come as a surprise to us.

Knowing that a hurricane is on the way doesn't really prepare you for the real thing.

Thursday 16 January
She is farting ten times more often. I'm not complaining, I'm just commenting. Because she is more sensitive to smells, I'm not allowed to fart at all. The books don't warn you about these vexations.

Cuddling on the sofa isn't so easy when there are three of you. 'I'm right on the edge,' she complained, even though I was flattened against the back.

We were watching a video of *Truly, Madly, Deeply*. Kate spent half the evening in tears, even making snorting pig noises at one point. It's about a dead man who comes back to comfort his mourning wife.

'It makes me think of you dying,' she said.

I saw the film about ten years ago. I enjoyed it again this time, but differently. The scene where the baby is born – 'A new life! A new life!' – seemed cloyingly sentimental a decade ago. Now it brought tears to my eyes. I pushed them back.

Our baby has been quiet for a couple of days. 'You must make more noise,' Kate told it.

Friday 17 January
Kate was huffing and puffing as she tried to put her tights on. It is getting harder for her to reach her feet.

'It's going to get bigger and bigger,' she said, staring at her stomach, grumpy-faced. As if she hasn't thought about this before. After weeks of saying that she is looking forward to having a big bump, she is starting to think that maybe it's not such a great thing.

Now she isn't so sure that going to Rome in March is a good idea. If she is this uncomfortable on her own sofa, what is she going to be like in a cheap airline seat? Will there be any pleasure sitting in a Roman café when she's got leg cramps? Italian food, which is God's gift to the world, is an instrument of torture when you're constipated.

Her tummy is hard. She can't sit still for long because her legs are restless. 'I'm worried,' she said. She can't feel the baby moving.

Saturday 18 January
Woke at 6.30 this morning. Couldn't get back to sleep so I got up, read a book, wrote something and even cleaned the kitchen floor. I watched the day brighten and warm until sunlight was pouring through the windows. The early hours of the morning had given me energy, clarity and a sense of

optimism. This is good, I decided. Getting up early means you get so much more from the day. When the baby is here and waking us at dawn, perhaps we'll be able to get more done.

By 9.15 am I was heavy-limbed and heavy-lidded and went back to bed for a nap.

Went to see a football match with friends this afternoon. Leyton Orient 2–Hull City 0. We sat among the Hull fans, who started off by singing 'I'm City till I die, City till I die.' They soon forgot this sentiment – they booed their team off the pitch at half-time. It was the first time in ages that I've felt carefree, unencumbered by the need to work, if only for a few hours.

Later I phoned Kate to see if she wanted to see a film. She decided that she ought to, since everyone says it will be impossible when the baby is here. At the Odeon on Shaftesbury Avenue we saw *The Good Girl*.

Today's lesson. You can't run for buses when you're pregnant. We walked through Trafalgar Square and waited for a number 12 bus to Peckham. Midnight came but the bus didn't. It was a freezing night. After half an hour, a large crowd of cold people had gathered. Finally a red Routemaster appeared at the end of Whitehall and stopped at traffic lights, just short of the bus stop. The English are famous for forming orderly queues, but this virtue seems to disappear from the national character below a certain temperature. Twenty people started running for the bus and forced their way on board before it had set off from the traffic lights. This Darwinian approach to bus travel meant that, when the bus halted at the bus stop, all the seats were occupied. Kate stepped on board, then the conductress stretched out an arm and blocked my path, declaring that there was only standing room available for one person. In fact there was room for several people, but the rules only allow five people to stand, and the conductress was eager to reassert her authority after the invasion at the traffic lights. I told Kate to go home ahead of me, but she didn't want to, and she was right, it wouldn't have been sensible for her to walk through Peckham on her own in the early hours. I wanted to shout out, 'All you people who just pushed onto the bus. You just stopped a pregnant woman getting home. Sleep well.' But I only thought about this later. We stepped off the bus into the cold. But there was a happy ending. Another bus appeared after two minutes, almost empty. We got the prized front seats on the top deck and had the pleasure of overtaking the previous bus on the way home.

Sunday 19 January Week 23

We woke up late. We were supposed to be meeting Kate's friends, Kathy and Pete, in a local café at 11.30. Waking up early on a Sunday morning isn't a problem for them because they have two babies. Following IVF treatment, they had twin boys a few months ago. 'Two for the price of one', as they put it.

Nice people, nice babies, nice breakfast. But I left feeling depressed. They described waking up four times last night to tend to the babies. They grab bowls of cornflakes and eat as quickly as possible whenever there's a brief hiatus in childcare duties. They confessed to feeling angry if they find their partner selfishly reading a newspaper for a few seconds.

Reading has become a luxury. Recently Pete read a short story about a father who drives his mother-in-law to the train station. It's a 20-minute round trip but he returns after 30 minutes. When he comes through the front door his wife accuses him – 'You've been reading, haven't you?' – and he has to admit that he stopped in a car park for ten minutes to read a book. This story made Pete laugh, the bitter laughter of recognition.

He is a journalist for the *Independent*. He says his brain has been reduced to functioning in a very basic 'primal state'. Kathy, trying to look on the bright side, said that he still has 'the odd thought'.

But they have given us hope that we will still be able to go to the cinema. They have been to The Big Scream, a weekly event at Clapham Picture House exclusively for parents with children under one year old. If a child starts crying during the film, a bottle or a nipple is shoved in its mouth. Apparently, most of the babies don't seem to mind the explosions and bright lights on the screen; for them the whole world is an adventure movie at the moment. The twins found the new James Bond movie tame compared to Clapham High Street.

Kathy says that one of the twins started choking on his vomit and stopped breathing for a second. Kathy hit him hard on the back to clear his airway, then phoned the health visitor to tell her what had happened. She said, 'I bashed him on the back.'

'You didn't bash him, you patted him,' said the health visitor.

'No, I bashed him.'

'No, you patted him.'

Kathy understood. If she admitted to 'bashing' her baby, the law would require the health visitor to report her to one of the child protection agencies.

Monday 20 January
During the night I turned over in bed and tried to cuddle Kate, but she fended me off apologetically. She pushed me away and then patted me as if to say that I shouldn't take it personally. 'I need space.' She couldn't get comfortable. She kept getting up to go to the toilet. Her stomach feels harder as the baby grows and grows and grows.

Last night in bed she could feel the baby's presence for the first time in a few days; she had 'the windy feeling' again. Then the baby was quiet all day until she sat down in a chair after supper, when she felt vague movements. Not satisfied with this, she started prodding herself. This was recommended by Kathy. When she was carrying her babies, she used to poke her stomach to get a reaction from them, just to reassure herself that they were alive.

Tuesday 21 January
Television is infested by DIY programmes. I hate them, not just because DIY is a tedious subject, but because the programmes encourage people to improve their homes. If you live in a London street, this means that there is always noise coming from someone's new patio or loft conversion. The man next door is constantly hammering or drilling something. Last week there was a choir of drills either side of our flat. This made it impossible to work, so I ended up working all night, and the drills stopped me sleeping during the day.

Now I'm wishing I'd paid more attention to those programmes. We have a list of things we need to do to the flat before the baby arrives. This week I've made a start. Putting grouting around the bath has taken me three days. It is noisy work. Every so often I shout 'Fucking hell!' as I discover more cracking or flaking.

To overcome my DIY deficiencies, I am seeking expert advice. This afternoon I popped into a bookshop when I was walking through Dulwich Village, hoping to sneak a look in a DIY manual, but there wasn't one in the entire shop. The people of Dulwich Village are too rich for DIY. All their house books are about interior design and architecture. It's the same story on the childcare shelves. I was looking for a medical reference book about children's health, but all I found was *The Good Nanny Guide*.

Kate keeps bursting into tears, but I'm trying not to take it personally. She got home from work at 8.10 pm. I told her off for working so late. I know I've been working until 5 am, but I'm not pregnant. She was grumpy all evening.

In bed, earlier this week, she pushed me away because she needed space. Tonight I gave her space and she asked for a cuddle.

She had a fit of crying. 'What's wrong?' 'I don't know.' Eventually she said that there's so much to do, work is stressful and she doesn't feel that she can cope. She is usually one of the most composed and capable people I know, so this crying fit was out of character, a bit like Boadicea suddenly announcing to her army that it's all too much and she needs a break.

I was on the verge of sleep when she said, 'Are you asleep?'

'No.'

'Put your hand here.'

I put my hand on her belly. For the first time, I felt the baby move, a soft thud in the palm of my hand. It was one of the nicest moments of my life.

Wednesday 22 January

All day I've been thinking about feeling the baby's kick last night.

This afternoon we went to the solicitor on Lordship Lane and signed our Last Will and Testament. If Kate dies, I get her flat. If I die, she gets my bicycle. The real reason for signing the wills was to ensure that our kids are entitled to inherit. As we left the offices of William Bailey, Kate gripped my arm. 'It feels like we've just got married,' she said.

We have started referring to 'our kids'. We seem to assume that we'll be having more than one. Now that we're in the 23rd week, we're more willing to put it into words, more confident that it's really going to happen.

When Kate cries these days I just put my arms round her. Sometimes I risk saying 'It's OK, it's OK' even though I don't usually know what 'it' is.

Thursday 23 January

She has heartburn, a fiery feeling in her oesophagus. And her constipation is having serious consequences. She blocked the toilet at work today.

In bed she read a short story that she read three days ago but has forgotten already. She says it's not because she's pregnant, it's because she's tired.

Friday 24 January

I've got a sore hip. Went to see an osteopath. A Canadian woman called Beverley. She told me that she has just returned to work after maternity leave; she gave birth to her second child five months ago. She has two boys. She told me, 'Work is what I do for a rest.'

This evening we went to see a radio programme being recorded. Making sure that mother and baby eat well means carrying emergency supplies if you're more than ten minutes away from your fridge. We took ham sandwiches with us and ate them on the bus. At the Oval we transferred to the Northern Line where she produced a packet of ginger cookies 'with no added sugar'. So she added her own sugar, a large bar of Green & Black's organic chocolate. When it comes from a health food shop and has the word 'organic' on the packet, chocolate doesn't seem such a vice. She was already looking forward to the next meal. 'We can eat pasta afterwards.'

The radio show included a useful childcare tip. One of the panellists has told his children that the musical greeting of an ice cream van indicates that it has run out of ice cream.

She was worried again tonight. 'I hope baby is all right, I haven't felt it moving.'

Saturday 25 January

'Many couples find that a position in which the woman is on top is more comfortable.' That's the opinion of the authors of *The Pregnancy Book*. They must have written that as a joke. In my experience, by this stage of pregnancy, if the pregnant woman goes on top, the man will have limited mobility and may not be able to do much more than twitch ineffectually.

I spent an hour painstakingly applying sealant around our bath and 20 minutes tearing it off again because I'd done it all wrong. The sticky white gunk looked like a rough sea.

As we approached the library in Peckham, a too-friendly woman came up to us and said, 'I just want you to know that Jesus loves you.' If Jesus really loved me, the library would've been open. Instead we went to our alternative local reference library, also known as W H Smith, where I read all about sealant. I resisted buying a book called *100 Things You Don't Need A Man For – The DIY Book for Women*. Back home, with a combination of increased knowledge and lower expectations, I achieved a result I could live with. That last sentence is probably a motto for parenthood.

In Mothercare we bought a book called *Baby & Child Healthcare* by, inevitably, Miriam Stoppard. This is an essential A–Z home reference to children's illnesses. I opened the book at random and saw Penis Caught in Zip. Glancing at the range of health catastrophes that children are prone to,

I realised that this is a book that every parent should buy but not read unless absolutely necessary.

Eddie says that he suffered from Penis Caught in Zip when he was six. His grandfather had to yank his foreskin out of the zip's teeth. He predicts that we will have a girl. The problem with boys, he tells me, is that they pee in your face.

The baby was moving again tonight. I felt a light thump against my thumb.

Sunday 26 January   Week 24

Planning for the future used to mean booking cinema tickets a day in advance. Now we're having to make big decisions based on huge assumptions. One reason Kate favours the Renault, she said today, is that we might have another baby in the next three years.

Pregnancy makes the future predictable and unpredictable; I'm not sure what's more daunting, the unforeseeable crises or the foreseeable drudgery.

Last night I was reading that the baby is sensitive to indicators of the mother's mood. If the mother is happy, the baby responds to the endorphins released into the bloodstream. If the mother is frightened, the baby responds to her adrenaline. If the mother is angry or miserable, the baby can sense changes in the pitch and tone of her voice and the tension in her body.

This evening we had evidence of our baby's sensitivity. We were inside Clapham Picture House watching Roman Polanski's film, *The Pianist*, about the fate of the Jewish community in Nazi-occupied Poland. The first hour was relentlessly brutal and barbaric. Kate leant over to me and said, 'The baby is moving a lot.' The film was disturbing all of us.

Monday 27 January

A friend looks me in the eye and gives me some sincere advice about fatherhood. 'Buy a digital camera.' He assures me that 90 per cent of the thousands of photographs we're obliged to take of our baby will be disappointing; a digital camera means we can erase these. As a father of two, he says that the greatest expense of parenthood – more than nappies and buggies etc – is photographic equipment.

Today we had an email from Finland where Kate's friends have had a baby. They have included a website address where we can view pictures of the entire family.

The impulse to document photographically every moment of your child's life reminds me of the *Santaland Diaries*, the autobiographical account by David Sedaris of the Christmas he was employed as an elf in Macy's department store in New York. As the official Photo Elf, he regularly witnessed desperate parents who, after queuing for over an hour, were determined not to leave without a photo of their son or daughter on Santa's lap, even if the child was terrified of Santa: 'Tonight I saw a woman slap and shake her sobbing daughter, yelling, "Goddamn it, Rachel, get on that man's lap and smile or I'll give you something to cry about!" I often take photographs of crying children.'

Kate calls me over. By the time I get there, the baby has stopped kicking. When I talk to the baby, Kate tells me off for tickling her belly button with my nose. She has heartburn, a burning feeling all the way down her throat.

Tuesday 28 January

Panic last night. Just for a moment. It was two in the morning. Couldn't sleep. An emotion got through my defences. I have a baby on the way. How am I going to survive? Fuck, fuck, fuck. I sent a text message to my useless producer, Ollie. He has a meeting tomorrow with a wealthy LA-based producer who says he wants to help us make the film. I wrote: 'Please get realistic prognosis from Edward S. When r we likely to film? Will he put money where his mouth is? Need money, not bullshit.'

Thinking about the baby makes me feel happier. The film business is an adult, tainted, grubby, dishonest thing. Whereas my child is new, pure, a reason for optimism. I know that a child will bring its own complications, but until it is born I can savour its redeeming innocence.

Kate and I were hugging. My hand was on her bottom. There seemed to be more of it.

She said: 'Is my bum bigger?'

'No.'

'Be honest.'

'Honestly, no.'

'Look me in the eyes. Is it bigger?'

'No.'

Wednesday 29 January

Not the most thrilling day of my life. But the pregnancy gives a sense of worth even to dull days. As a writer, I'm busy but often feel that I'm not actually getting anywhere. As an expectant father, I'm not actually doing much, yet I feel that every day is progress.

Kate came home from work with a craving for Yorkshire puddings, so we had them for supper. I asked her, 'What did you have for lunch?'

'Yorkshire puddings.'

It's nearly the end of January. Time to review the progress I've made with my New Year's resolution to improve my cooking. Marks out of ten? Zero. Absolutely nothing has changed. Must do better. Must do something.

'Ow!'

'What?'

'I just got one of those twinges.'

When she bends down, she gets shooting pains in her buttocks.

Her belly is squishy, like a balloon filled with water. I felt the baby kick again. It made me feel ridiculously happy. What an amazing thing. A life is growing in there. I am awestruck. My mind is boggled. A baby restores your sense of wonder.

Thursday 30 January

Kate peed herself this morning. She was standing in the hall when she dribbled down her leg.

I popped into Mothercare on impulse as I was passing, just to look around. This isn't something I've ever done before. I read an entertaining book called *The Very Hungry Caterpillar*. And there was a book incorporating a battery-operated microphone so that you can record yourself (and your child, who will probably want a go as well) making cow and sheep noises and then you can play them back. There's a lot to look forward to.

Blustery snow, not enough to settle. Minus nine degrees in the gales. Our boiler, which provides heating and hot water, has broken down again. A man came round recently to assess the cost of a replacement. He said a new boiler will cost £2,248.82. Another company has quoted us £1,300.

We went to sleep at 11 pm, cuddling together for warmth. I woke up at 2.45 am and got out of bed. Couldn't sleep. Worked until 6.45 am, then went back to bed for a couple of hours.

Friday 31 January

We had a scare today.

A bright cold morning. The air bit my ears as we strode, slid, scurried across snow and ice to the hospital for our second ultrasound scan. We were looking forward to seeing the baby again.

The sonographer was a young woman called Caitlin. She squirted the gel on Kate's stomach. Kate screamed because it was so cold. We all smiled.

At first Caitlin had trouble getting a good view of the baby because it was lying with its head down. The baby seemed fragmented, a gathering of dark blobs and grey balloons which occasionally coalesced into a recognisable shape: a nose all on its own, a floating hand, a disembodied leg, a snaking spine, the pulsing chambers of the heart. Its foot was up near its head; it seemed to be kissing its toe. Eventually we saw a good view of the skull and the brain. The circumference of the skull was a thick line; the brain was a grey blob.

On one side, between the brain's mass and the skull's arc, there was a zeppelin-shaped blackness.

I said, 'What's that big gap between the brain and the skull? Is that normal?'

Caitlin said, 'I'm just measuring it. I'll be able to tell you if it comes within the normal range.'

There were certain measurements she couldn't make because the baby was in the wrong position. She asked Kate to lie on her side. The baby was stubborn and refused to move. Caitlin suggested that we should walk up and down the corridor for a while and give the baby time to change position. Kate offered to eat some chocolate; she has been told that the sweetness makes the baby move. Caitlin said, 'Yes, I've heard midwives say that. I don't know, I'm not a midwife, but you can try it.' So we went to the corridor and ate chocolate. I read three books. *Little Pup. Pooh's First Songs. Guess How Much I Love You.*

Back in the darkened room, we looked at the screen. Caitlin told us that there seemed to be 'a little extra fluid around the brain'. If we didn't mind, she was going to ask us to wait outside again until a consultant was able to see us. They wanted to scan the baby with a more accurate machine. So we sat in the waiting room.

'Do you want your book?' asked Kate.

'OK.'

I held the novel in front of my face. After a couple of minutes, she turned to look at me and caught me not reading. I was staring through the page. I felt hollow. Then there was a weight in my stomach and in the back of my skull. It was dread.

After half an hour, we were called into another room. Kate lay down again, resting the back of her head on her arm so that she could see the images on the screen. I held her hand.

Jorge was from Brazil. He was supervising Maria, who was from Cyprus, as she operated the scanner. It was a new machine, which provided clearer images than the other one and allowed greater magnification. While Maria took new measurements, Jorge chatted to us amiably. 'Do you want a boy or a girl?' We said that we didn't want to know. He persisted. 'But if you had two buttons in front of you now, green and purple, green for a boy and purple for a girl, which one would you press?' Kate said she really didn't mind.

I said, 'Purple.'

'A good answer,' said Maria.

As Maria operated the machine, Jorge kept leaning over and interfering, pushing levers, twisting buttons, adjusting her hand as it angled the scanning device over Kate's tummy. I have a friend just like him, who manages to be likeable and annoying at the same time. After a while, Maria stood up, sick of his interference.

'You finish,' she said.

'No,' he protested, but she had already vacated the seat. He sat down and took control of the machine.

'What jobs do you do?' he asked us. Kate said that she was a psychologist. 'That's nice,' he said. I said that I was a playwright. 'That's nice,' he said. We already knew that he was an obstetrician so Kate asked him for his opinion about water births. 'They are a mess,' he said, 'a complete mess. There is blood and bodily fluids everywhere. It is a nice way to give birth, but it is a mess.' He was charming but I wished he would shut up. I was trying to concentrate on the details on the monitor.

There it was again, a black vacuum between the baby's brain and the skull.

But I was wrong. Jorge explained that the blackness wasn't a void. The zeppelin-shaped hole wasn't a hole at all. It was fluid. Our baby appears to have a slightly enlarged ventricle, he told us.

'In its heart?' I asked, confused.

'No, in its brain.'

I didn't know that there were ventricles in the brain. In fact, they are present on both sides of the brain and they produce a fluid that oozes down the spine during foetal development. These ventricles are 7 millimetres long on average. Anything up to 10 millimetres is considered normal. Our baby's ventricle measures 10½ millimetres on this machine. On the previous machine it had been measured as 12 millimetres. 'It is not very serious,' Jorge told us. I felt slightly relieved, not fully convinced.

Soon a cardiologist arrived. He didn't even look at Kate or me. He stared at the monitor, declared that our baby's heart was normal, and left without acknowledging us.

'This is just a routine precaution,' said Jorge. 'We check the baby's heart and spine to make sure that everything is normal.'

He gave us a guided tour of our baby, zooming in on its face. We saw our baby yawn and waggle its tongue. Our baby has an upturned nose. Jorge mentioned that he could see the palate.

I said, 'Can you see the palate?' I hadn't even thought about asking. I was born with a cleft lip and palate and I've been concerned that my baby might be born with one. This machine revealed the baby's face and most of the palate; the only thing it can't detect is the soft palate at the back of the mouth.

'This baby does not have a cleft lip,' said Jorge. And the part of the palate that was visible appeared normal.

Doctors don't really know what causes cleft lip and palate, but it's believed that there can be a genetic factor. I was so delighted that I hadn't passed this on to my baby. Tears welled up. I fought them back. I was glad the room was dark. I couldn't speak for a few minutes.

Now there is something else to worry about instead. We were joined by Janet, one of the senior consultants, who scanned Kate's stomach for the umpteenth time. Our baby's condition, Janet explained, is called ventriculomegaly. It is a borderline case. It is just beyond the limits of what is considered a normal measurement. Sometimes the condition is accompanied by other abnormalities – for example, there can be indications of spina bifida. But our baby appears to be perfectly normal.

Janet told us to come back to the hospital in two weeks for another scan to make sure that the condition is not progressive; that is, to measure the length of the ventricle to see if it has increased. If it has, there is a 5 per cent chance that our baby will have a developmental disability. This can be physical or mental. It could be a weakness in one leg, or it could mean that our child has a slightly lower IQ.

The other implication of ventriculomegaly is that the likelihood of having a baby with Down's syndrome has doubled. Now the probability is estimated to be 1 in 629. Janet said that, if we feel that we need to know for certain, we have the option of an amniocentesis.

We've been offered this before. It involves putting a needle through the mother's abdomen to extract some of the amniotic fluid surrounding the baby so that it can be tested for signs of spina bifida, Down's syndrome or other genetic disorders. This procedure carries a 1 per cent risk of miscarriage. Kate said, glancing at me, 'Well, we'll have to talk about it, but I don't want that.'

I said, 'No, I don't think that's necessary.'

'Any questions?' said Janet.

Kate asked if there was a risk of hydrocephalus. This is when a blockage of the fluid causes a build-up of pressure inside the skull, potentially causing brain damage and a malformed head.

'No,' said Janet, 'your baby does not have hydrocephalus.' She also assured us that all the evidence suggests that multiple scans have no adverse effect on the foetus or the mother.

We arranged an appointment for another scan in two weeks. On Valentine's Day.

Just what we didn't need. In addition to all our irrational fears. Rational fears.

As we left the room with two printed images of our baby, Jorge stopped us at the door and said teasingly, 'The pictures are very typical of that sex.' We laughed.

We had spent four hours in the hospital. Kate works in another hospital across the road. We went to have lunch in the canteen there and bumped into two of her colleagues, Craig and Gemma. They were sympathetic and suggested that modern pregnancy is over-medicalised. They have a point. Not all hospitals in the UK offer a second scan at 20+ weeks. We would never have known about this potential abnormality and we would've been spared all this fear.

We are getting upset about half a millimetre. It seems a very mathematical approach to the creation of life. It occurs to me that there's a similarity between writing and pregnancy. In the film business, producers try to reduce the creative process to a series of rules about structure and they judge a script by numbers (of acts, of pages, of characters, of bums on seats, of dollars). In pregnancy, the doctors analyse a baby's development also with mathematical measurements (of limbs, of organs, of ventricles), which propagate the misleading impression that the variations and mysteries of creation can be confined to narrow scientific formulae. Life, like art, cannot be reduced to numbers.

Kate went to work in the afternoon. I met a friend at the NFT where we watched *Persona*, a bleak Ingmar Bergman film, which came as light relief after the morning's trauma. In the evening, to celebrate Chinese New Year, we met other friends and stood next to the Thames to watch a dragon made out of fireworks. That's what it was meant to be. It was just a long string of minor explosions spiralling around the Millennium Bridge and climbing up the chimney of Tate Modern. Afterwards there was supposed to be jasmine tea and fortune cookies inside the vast art gallery, but the fireworks had set off the fire alarms so the building had to be evacuated. We all went to Chinatown and ate too much. A couple of friends asked about the baby, so we mentioned that the scan had revealed a minor abnormality. Nothing serious, I said. We hopped off the number 12 bus on Rye Lane and walked home, chatting about trivia.

In bed, Kate sobbed. We cuddled the baby. Kate says she hasn't felt it move since the scan. I wish it could be born now so I could give it a hug and a kiss. All I want is for it to have a fair chance.

Saturday 1 February
Kate got angry with the shower this morning. The water wouldn't stay at the right temperature.

'Baby's not moving at all,' she said.

'I promise you the baby will kick.'

Later, the baby kicked twice.

We went for a walk around Peckham Rye. I said, 'I have a feeling that everything will be fine.'

'I have a feeling that it won't.'

'Is that a feeling or a fear?'

'It's hard to tell the difference.'

We discussed whether to tell our friends about the results of the scan. Kate is inclined to tell people. I would prefer to keep the news to ourselves.

I don't want people's interest and sympathy.

For supper we were invited to the house of a Scottish friend to celebrate Burns' Night, even though it isn't Burns' Night. They asked about the baby. We didn't tell them about the results of the scan, partly because other friends there announced that they are planning to get married in May and we didn't want to piss on their bonfire.

We ate haggis and read poems out loud. Our hostess produced her deepest Scots accent and I only understood one word in ten. Fortunately, the rules were relaxed and we were allowed to read the work of any poet. Kate found a poem by Sheenagh Pugh called 'Sometimes' whose optimism appealed to me:

> Sometimes things don't go, after all,
> from bad to worse. Some years, muscadel
> faces down frost; green thrives, the crops don't fail,
> sometimes a man aims high, and all goes well.
>
> A people sometimes will step back from war;
> elect an honest man; decide they care
> enough, that they can't leave some stranger poor.
> Some men become what they were born for.
>
> Sometimes our best efforts do not go
> amiss; sometimes we do as we meant to.
> The sun will sometimes melt a field of sorrow
> that seemed hard frozen: may it happen for you.

Sunday 2 February   **Week 25**

I'm not feeling so optimistic any more. I typed *ventriculomegaly* into an internet search engine.

> Ventriculomegaly has been associated with other abnormalities, such as of the brain, kidneys and heart.

I wasn't too worried when I read this because our baby was checked thoroughly and appeared to be anatomically normal. Then I read the next sentence.

Up to 10% of these other abnormalities are not detectable by prenatal ultrasound ... the most common concurrent anomaly is spina bifida ... enlargement of the lateral ventricles is associated with schizophrenia and other neurodevelopmental disorders ...

Information is not the same as knowledge. You have to be careful about using the web to research health information. It can turn you into a cyberchondriac.

Only one thing is clear. We're going to be spending a lot more time in hospital.

The fetus is followed with serial ultrasounds. If the ventriculomegaly is stable, the fetus is carried to term.

I wasn't sure if reading all this stuff was helpful, but I persisted anyway.

Observation of fetal ventriculomegaly offers our best opportunity to detect malformation of the CNS (central nervous system). Ventriculomegaly is the "tip of the iceberg" (of anomalous CNS development) that we seek.

With all my heart I am hoping that there is no iceberg. I read dozens of obfuscatory academic articles from medical journals. I read articles that gave me hope:

... those with mild isolated ventriculomegaly of less than 12mm have an excellent prognosis ... in ten cases, the scan showed mild unilateral ventriculomegaly with an atrium width between 11 and 13mm and this remained stable up to term ... No obvious cause was found and the outcome was normal in all cases.

The problem is that doctors don't agree with each other. The cold, clumsy prose of the medical literature gives conflicting accounts of the longer-term prospects. I read articles that took hope away:

MVM is associated with a similarly broad range and prevalence (78%) of serious concomitant anomalies. Further, overall mortality of fetuses with MVM is strikingly high (75%) and comparable with that for fetuses with all degrees of ventriculomegaly. Impressively, this poor outcome was noted despite the absence of severe CNS malformations such as holoprosencephaly or hydranencephaly. Finally, the prognosis of survivors with MVM is relatively poor. At least 25% of living neonates are significantly handicapped or likely to be so.

It is clear that the prospects are calamitous if the ventricle becomes progressively wider or if other symptoms of abnormality are detected in future scans. Now I am hoping that our baby is a boy because there is some evidence that the presence of large ventricles in males is less likely to have sinister implications.

> A large retrospective study showed that male fetuses had a slightly larger atrial size ... A large proportion of mild and stable cases in large-for-dates and/or male fetuses are likely to represent a variation of the normal fetal anatomy.

I wanted to ignore the pessimistic data and to focus on the hopeful statistics and the stories with happy endings. If I could find them. Much of the medical literature seems to suggest that we should prepare for the worst. Some articles left me deeply depressed. Stubbornly, I kept searching the websites. I was looking for hope. I found it in an article whose statistics seemed more optimistic:

> 90% of fetuses with a lateral ventricular measurement of 10 to 11mm will be normal after birth and this measurement probably represents a normal variant in males ... Overall, the majority of fetuses with isolated mild ventriculomegaly have a good prognosis.

I am choosing to believe this. It gives us a 90 per cent chance of a healthy baby.

Despite all the advantages of technology and medicine, our baby's future is unknowable. The internet has given me more questions than answers. After all my research I am left clinging to this one hope ... that our baby will be lucky.

I was still reading when Kate got back from her antenatal yoga class. I hid the page. I didn't tell her what I'd found. She knows where the information is, if she wants it. She didn't mention the subject all day, so I didn't. I tried not to be too gloomy or tetchy, and probably failed. We discussed banal things like towel rails.

Fiddling with the remote control, I found myself accidentally watching *Songs of Praise*. There was an interview with a middle-aged couple who've adopted a disabled child. The parents were saying how wonderful the experience is. I admire them, but I don't think I'm like them. I don't want a severely disabled child. But that's the risk we're taking.

I am ashamed of these feelings, but I can't deny they're there.

None of the pregnancy books has much to say about specific abnormalities that may be detected by the ultrasound. The woman who wrote *The Rough Guide to Pregnancy & Birth* reflects, 'The scan left me feeling happier and more relaxed than I can remember.'

In the evening Kate dozed off while lying on the sofa. When she awoke, she was too tired to lift herself up; she was pinned down by her own stomach. I had to haul her up.

Monday 3 February
According to research mentioned on the radio, by now 50 per cent of people have abandoned their New Year's resolutions. This prompted me to make a start on one of mine. I told Kate that my New Year's resolution was to improve my cooking. She admits that she isn't giving me a chance. She comes home with particular cravings and starts cooking straight away; she hasn't got the patience to watch me faffing around with kitchen utensils. This evening she graciously allowed me to cook pasta with broccoli and pesto and cheese.

She looked glum.

'What?'

'I've been having morbid thoughts about the baby.'

So I told her that I've been reading about ventriculomegaly. I only mentioned my more hopeful findings. I told her that our baby's measurement is only just outside the normal range, and 10½ millimetres is natural and healthy for some foetuses, especially if they're boys. She said, 'Maybe we should find out what sex it is.' I've had the same thought. If our baby is a boy, there's more chance that the size of the ventricle is innocuous.

Eric phoned. Kate told him about the scan and said that one of the measurements in the brain was 'at the higher end of the average range … it could just mean that some babies have larger ventricles than others'. We are trying to be optimistic.

Eric's young daughter has heart problems. Last week the little girl turned blue and they had to rush her to hospital. The parents aren't sleeping at all. People talk about having kids and settling down, but it's the most unsettling thing you can do.

'Baby hasn't moved all day,' she reported. I told her not to worry.

We don't often listen to music. I suggested that we should listen to a CD, because it's something the baby can share with us. It's something we can do together, the three of us. It made me feel like I was doing something for the baby. I suggested Van Morrison or Joni Mitchell. Kate chose Debussy and Vivaldi. It's not my favourite music. But the baby seemed to like it. It kicked and kicked.

Tuesday 4 February

In *A Life's Work*, Rachel Cusk refers to '… the drama of which childbirth is merely the opening scene'.

In fact, the drama begins long before the birth. Life has begun already. Kate says paediatricians count age from the moment of conception for the baby's first year. So when a child born 2 weeks premature is 2 weeks old, in a paediatrician's eyes it is 40 weeks old. Our baby is already a little person. I am already its father. I feel love and responsibility for this tiny individual struggling to grow.

I sent copies of the scan pictures to Warrington in an envelope addressed to 'Nana and Grandad'. I thought twice about writing that. What if our baby dies before it is born? It's possible. Maybe I shouldn't implicate its grandparents in the situation any more than they already are? I might simply be increasing the pain they will feel if things don't work out. I had this thought but dismissed it. You can't live like that. We have to embrace life rather than keep it at arm's length. I know people who live their lives self-protectively, trying not to get too close to anything they might lose. The fear of loss, ironically, means they are losing out.

Kate was panicked by her belly button tonight. Over the weeks it has become bigger, stretched, a yawning cave. Now it has closed again; shrivelled and wrinkled, it's back to looking like my gran's mouth when she hasn't got her teeth in. 'Have I shrunk?' asked Kate. An answer came to me. 'No, your skin has stretched, that's all.' She wasn't convinced. She said, 'Let's measure it.' So we uncoiled the tape measure and wrapped it around her abdomen at the level of the belly button. The last time we did this, two and a half weeks ago, the circumference of her waist measured 93 centimetres. Today it measures 97 centimetres. So we felt reassured.

Later, getting ready for bed, we noticed that the bump has moved and changed shape; it seems to hang lower as if the baby is heavier, more substantial. 'It's suddenly got big!' she said happily.

Her farts are noxious. The pregnancy books don't warn you about this. Reading in bed, we've perfected a technique of tucking the sheets around our bodies so any odours can't escape.

Mike Barker, the film director, phoned. They can't cast Dougray Scott any more because his name doesn't attract enough finance. It did a year ago, apparently, but not now. So the script is being sent to other actors. Ralph Fiennes first of all. If he doesn't like it, they want to send it to Kenneth Branagh. Six years of writing and waiting and everything depends on whether a couple of actors feel like doing it.

I had to look. In a newsgroup I came across an encouraging letter from one parent to another:

> Re: borderline ventriculomegaly. Posted on August 10 at 07:54:33:
>
> Hi, I was in your situation a year ago exactly. When I was 20 wks pg, the doctors found multiple problems on US, including mild bilateral ventriculomegaly (10–12 mm), bilateral choroid plexus cysts, dilated kidneys, echogenic foci in the heart. Amnio was normal. We had follow-up US every 4 wks. It was the worst thing I ever went through. Anyway, my son was born at 37 wks completely healthy. He is now 6 mos and developing 100% normally. Like I said, it was the worst time in my life, and I am so blessed now to have a healthy boy. I will never forget that horror. I think more and more babies are being diagnosed with borderline ventriculomegaly as ultrasound technology improves. Hope this helps, Judith

A strange thing. I put the images from last week's ultrasound scan in a photograph album next to the images from the first scan. At the time, we thought those first images were wonderfully exciting and well defined. We couldn't understand why other people weren't as impressed by them as we were. Now our opinion of them has changed completely. They seem blurred, grey and indistinct compared to the new images.

Wednesday 5 February

On Piccadilly I visited the huge Waterstone's bookshop, which I often use as a reference library. All the books here are immaculate new editions, and no other London library has sofas and a café. I made my way to the medical section, searched the paediatric shelves and was shocked when I opened a book about children's ailments at a random page. There were colour photographs of dead and deformed children, including the ruptured back of an infant with spina bifida and the naked corpse of a child with anencephaly, which is when the top half of the head is missing or distorted. There were descriptions of hydrocephalus but not much about ventriculomegaly. I learnt about the function of the ventricles and the cerebrospinal fluid and the things that can go wrong. I'm not sure if I'm doing myself any favours by reading all this stuff. But if there are difficult choices ahead, I want to make them from a position of understanding.

Absurdly, I went from paediatrics to cosmetics. I wanted to buy a couple of board games as birthday presents for friends, so I went to the department stores on Oxford Street. As soon as you enter, you have to navigate through the cosmetic counters, trying not to inhale the choking cocktail of perfumes. The female members of staff ('Fragrance Advisors') have stiff hair and plucked orange faces. So do the male members of staff.

People were polite. I held the door open and they smiled and said, 'Thanks.' They held doors open for me and I smiled and said, 'Thanks.' But I felt emotionally dislocated all day, weighed down and close to tears. I kept having stupid thoughts. Our child's funeral. The consequences of disability. I told myself not to be so doom-laden.

In Selfridges I found the games department and, appropriately, ended up buying a board game called Cranium.

On the way home, I told myself that the baby will be born perfectly healthy if the traffic lights don't turn red before the bus goes past. The traffic lights turned amber. What does that mean? I forced myself to disembark from this foolish train of thought.

I went to a football match at the Den with a friend who is a Southampton fan. There were only 10,000 people in the stadium because most Millwall supporters are in jail. We were searched on the way into the ground. In my bag I had a flask of tea, bulky enough to conceal a weapon or to be used as one. The burly steward eyed me suspiciously. 'What's that?' 'Camomile tea,' I said feebly. This answer was so pathetic that he decided I was harmless, and let me in. The final score was Millwall 1–Southampton 2 after extra time in the FA Cup fourth-round replay. I can't really afford it, but all the thoughts of death have made me feel like living. A game of football, with its laughable self-importance, is a pleasing distraction from the rest of life.

Thursday 6 February
Got a text message from my mum: 'thankyou 4 the beautiful scans they r wonderful so beautiful i am lost 4 words luv as always xxx'.

I showed this to Kate, thinking she would be touched, and she laughed. 'It's not that beautiful! It looks like an alien.'

Kate isn't as worried about our baby's prospects as I am. Unlike me, she hasn't frightened herself by reading medical books. Last night she lay awake for three hours, worrying about the things she is going to miss at work when she is on maternity leave. But she was cheerful tonight when she rubbed her belly and thought about the baby. 'It's exciting!' she said.

Earlier, she had phoned from work sounding pleased. 'Baby's been moving all morning! Some people have noticed that I've had a growth spurt. Although it might just be that they notice it more because I'm wearing different clothes.'

We know it's growing, but what is growing? I am haunted by the photos of deformed babies.

Friday 7 February
'The way to love anything is to realise that it might be lost,' wrote G K Chesterton.

I've leant the pictures of our baby against the wall next to my desk. There's a snapshot of the foetus in – unsurprisingly – a foetal position. And a close-up of its head in profile. The face has an expression of innocent curiosity. In profile, our baby looks like Charlie Brown.

'I look forward to hugging it,' said Kate last night.

'I know, I wish I could do it now.'

We're going to Bristol for the weekend. Friends picked us up and we set off through London to the M4, listening to music that made the baby kick. The Van Morrison Effect. Along the way we stopped at motorway services for something to eat. About 30 miles from Bristol, all the traffic came to a halt. There were no vehicles on the other carriageway. We waited for an hour without moving. People got out of their cars to stretch their legs and talk. The man driving the car in front got out and urinated behind his front door. Kate did her pelvic floor exercises in the fast lane of the M4.

Sirens wailed as ambulances and police cars sped along the empty carriageway. There was a rumour that cars had crashed into the central reservation. Eventually the police told everyone to reverse, turn around and drive the wrong way along the motorway to the previous exit. We followed a minor road and rejoined the motorway beyond the crash scene.

Saturday 8 February

To arrive is a better thing than to travel hopefully. When I was 22 years old, I was run over by a lorry. I was cycling from London to Switzerland with a friend. The holiday wasn't a total success. We'd pedalled 20 miles along the A2 when I was hit by a lorry that was turning left at traffic lights. The impact knocked me on to the road. The lorry passed over me, its rear wheels rolling either side of my sprawled body. My bike was crushed. I was left with a broken jaw and a fractured cheekbone, cuts and bruises, and deafness and tinnitus in one ear. The lorry driver didn't even contact the hospital to ask if I was alive or dead. I've often reflected on the unfortunate convergence of our lives. I had cycled from south London that morning; he had driven from Lancaster. If I hadn't delayed my departure by a day, if one of us had set off a few minutes earlier or later, if one of us had been detained by traffic lights … then it would never have happened. We are at the mercy of ifs.

On the news we learnt that three vehicles were involved in last night's motorway crash. Two cars and a campervan burst into flames. One woman died.

The accident happened at 9.45 pm. We turned up at 10.30 pm after spending 45 minutes eating. If we hadn't stopped for food, we might've missed the traffic jam and got to Bristol on time. Or we might've been caught up in the crash. Maybe the leek and mushroom pie saved my life.

We're staying with old friends who have two little kids. On the stairs I met Melissa who'd had a dramatic night. Two of her teeth fell out. So far she has lost six teeth. She wants to lose eight teeth because her friend Belinda has lost eight teeth.

The six adults and two children intermingled throughout the day, continuing conversations from months ago when we last saw each other, adding the new stories from our lives. Kate asked me if I'd told anyone. No, I hadn't. Neither had she. We don't want to spoil the mood.

Later we showed the scans of our child. Everyone agreed that our baby looks like Charlie Brown. Our friends showed scans of their children. The image of their eldest daughter resembles the five-year-old she has become.

Kate's belly feels bigger but not heavier, she says. 'I keep stroking it, all the time. Can't help it.'

Sunday 9 February   **Week 26**
My friends asked me if I'm looking forward to having a baby. I said, 'Yes, it's exciting.' I could hear the lack of enthusiasm in my voice. It's because I am fearful of the type of child that's going to enter our lives. It was hard to match my friends' excitement. They're assuming it's going to be a normal, healthy child and I can't assume that any more.

In bed I did something useful. I scratched her back. It's one of the perks of pregnancy, I scratch her back and she doesn't have to scratch mine.

I asked her, 'How are you feeling about Friday?'

'OK, really. I feel as if it's going to be all right. It's growing. How do you feel?'

'I'm optimistic that it'll all be fine,' I lied. I'm not so sure.

We're sleeping in the attic room, an inverted V, like a large tent.

It's not just babies who wake you up during the night. So do expectant mothers. In the darkest hours, I was awoken by the patter of large feet. It was Kate trying to open the window to get more air.

The pace and weight of her breathing told me that she had gone straight back to sleep, which was annoying because I couldn't. I lay there for two hours, thinking about everything.

One of my friends in Bristol was trying to have kids. Then her husband, a lovely man in his mid-30s, died of cancer.

There's an old joke. How do you make God laugh? Tell him about your future plans.

Monday 10 February
I spent another couple of hours researching MVM so that I know which questions to ask on Friday. One complicating factor I've noticed in the medical literature is the temptation for doctors to exaggerate the severity of a problem in order to increase their chances of getting a research grant. One researcher, who had already received a $4,000 grant, stated that the number of foetuses with isolated MVM who had postnatal neurological

defects was 'a small but significant fraction'. Whereas a researcher who had not yet completed his study wrote about 'high risk for developmental delays' and said sweepingly 'it is hypothesized that fetuses with MVM will have significant neurocognitive abnormalities'. I hypothesise that in medicine, like in journalism, there is a temptation for investigators to overdramatise their findings in order to get attention. It's difficult for the reader not to be frightened by tabloid medicine.

After all my reading, the only thing I know is that the future is uncertain. In the absence of facts, there are fears.

There's evidence of a growth surge. Kate has had to widen her maternity trousers by several buttons to accommodate her stomach, which is bulging like a hot-air balloon.

This evening I cooked pasta with onions and courgettes. She asked for more, which I regard as a personal triumph. I don't think she has ever asked for more of my food.

She spoke to her mum who mentioned that Holly, Kate's niece, is getting cheeky and wilful. Holly is advanced for her age, Kate said proudly. This pride worries me. It makes me wonder how painful it will be if our own child isn't so bright and articulate.

Tonight Kate said we should write down some questions to ask on Friday. So I showed her the list of questions I've already compiled. We discussed what to do if the doctors suggest an MRI scan. Kate can't see the point. Only evidence of a terrible disorder that left the baby with no quality of life, she said, would make her consider a termination. Otherwise, there seems no good reason to submit herself and the baby to repeated scanning.

Tuesday 11 February
After work I met Kate in Brixton and we ate noodles. We missed a bus so we decided to walk home, a distance of three miles. We forget that we can't do things like we used to. Kate's pace got slower and slower but she made it back to Peckham.

Kate has a new party trick. When she blows her nose, she pees.

We discussed whether we want to know the baby's sex after all. I thought for a long time and said 'yes'. If we know that it's a boy, we'll have less cause to worry because it's more likely that the large ventricle is a normal feature of a male foetus. Kate said 'yes' immediately and for less tortured reasons. She said that she is impatient and curious to know if it's a boy or a girl. She has a hunch that it's a boy, she said, because she thinks she saw some testicles during the last scan.

I said to her, 'You seem calm about it all. Are you?'

'More than I was. I feel as if everything's going to be all right.'

Wednesday 12 February

Kate was working at home this afternoon. We went to the shops for vegetables and tea bags. We came home with vegetables, tea bags, a skirt and a blouse.

The government has warned Londoners to be 'alert but not alarmed' because of threats from terrorists.

I met a friend of a friend who asked me if I'm worried about bringing a baby into the world. I'm not. I quite like being alive and don't see why my child won't.

Some people, offering a reason for their reluctance or refusal to breed, say that this world is too cruel to inflict on a child. Others say that a child is too cruel to inflict on the world; the planet is already suffering from the presence of six billion humans, so why add to the problems?

I hope my child will be one of the nicer people. The way we live our lives affects the people around us. There are people who, on the whole, make the world a better place. And there are people who, on the whole, make the world a worse place. The world needs a continuing supply of the former to counteract the ceaseless supply of the latter. Even if our children don't manage to invent a cure for cancer, I still think there is some virtue in just being a decent human being.

Thursday 13 February

Went to visit my friend, Angela, in her new flat in East Dulwich. I witnessed the impossibility of getting a three-year-old to eat all his broccoli.

Angela recently organised a get-together for the mothers from her son's playgroup. Of the eight women, six of them are already separated or divorced from their children's father. Including Angela. Her husband lives abroad. She admits now that she used to cry herself to sleep every night.

These people are further along the road we've just turned on to. We're hoping for better luck on our journey.

On Lordship Lane I bought tulips for Kate, shades of purple and pink and red. In a shop on Northcross Road I ended up buying two cards because I couldn't decide which one I preferred. The woman behind the counter gave me a funny look, clearly suspicious of my reasons for buying two Valentine cards.

I was invited to have supper in Walthamstow with John and Ian. I knew it was a risk. John has many talents but cooking is not one of them. Compared to him, I'm Delia Smith. It was like going to a dinner party hosted by Stan Laurel. He plopped the tepid food onto the plates and then we had to wait five minutes while he cleared the dining table of his computer and printer. 'What are the crunchy bits?' I asked as I worked my way through the tagliatelle. 'Uncooked pasta,' he confessed. The pasta had the texture of conkers. It was *mal dente*. Then the back of Ian's wooden dining chair came apart.

Ian's wife is expecting a baby in April. They've been through worse things than we have. They were pregnant once before but lost the baby in the eighth week. This time the first scan revealed a cyst on his wife's ovary, so she was scanned repeatedly until it went away.

Our scan is tomorrow. At last. This week's social distractions have relieved the anxiety, but I'm still desperate to know what's going on in there.

Friday 14 February

Kate spoke to her uncle this morning, a neonatal specialist. He told her that King's is 'the best hospital in the country for cases of ventriculomegaly'. People come from all over the world to work and study in the obstetric department there. It is possibly the only place in the UK that has collected sufficient data to know what a 'normal range' of ventricle measurements is. We're lucky that it's our local hospital.

Or are we? Maybe the scans are making us worry needlessly. Many other hospitals around the country don't even offer a second scan. And, in the absence of reliable data, many doctors wouldn't have picked up on a borderline case like our baby's. This is the risk with ultrasound monitoring. It can detect serious treatable anomalies, or it can just make you worried about things that turn out to be untreatable or unimportant.

I met Kate in the waiting room of the hospital's new maternity building. She had come straight from work and I found her reading *The Handbook of Child & Adolescent Psychotherapy*. The other pregnant women in the room must've thought she was an over-keen prospective parent.

As usual it was a very London waiting room. A Muslim woman with her body and head covered in black fabric was sitting near a hippie woman whose curly brown and 'blonde' hair was exploding from her skull and whose reddish-pink blouse was cut low to reveal a black bra strap and eye-catching breasts. One woman was dressed for the Middle Ages and the other was dressed for a 1972 Rolling Stones concert. Nine out of ten women were accompanied by a man. One man had come prepared for a long wait; he was on page 3 of a 600-page Stephen King blockbuster.

After two hours we were called into the scanning room. A curtain was pulled across but the door was left open. People kept walking in and out to fiddle with the computer or to shuffle papers or to discuss the kidney of a patient who was waiting in the next room. It was as private as the lobby of an international hotel.

Kate's stomach was gelled and scanned by a trainee operator. His badge said his name was Jamal and he was based at the School of Medicine here. He wasn't very adept at scanning. He was trying to show us our baby's face but it was like staring at a blizzard.

'Look, there are the nostrils, the eyes. Would you like a picture of that?' said Jamal kindly, and we said yes because we didn't want to hurt his feelings. He printed a picture which, even later when we were able to scrutinise it, we couldn't recognise as human.

I knew from the last scan that it's important to keep the central channel of the brain horizontal on the screen. Jamal didn't seem to know this. I forced myself to appear more patient than I was feeling.

Jamal was supervised by a stocky man with a central European accent who eventually corrected the positioning of the scanner on Kate's belly. They asked us if we knew what sex our baby is and we said no. A beautiful, slim, short-skirted Greek woman (the kind of woman who shouldn't be allowed on a maternity ward where she probably induces waves of resentment in pregnant women who've just lost their waist) joined us and asked the same questions. No, we repeated, we don't know what sex our baby is.

'Do you know why we're asking?' said the Greek woman.

'Because large ventricles are more common in boys.'

'Yes,' said the Greek woman.

'But that's not a rule,' said Jamal.

Kate asked them, 'Do you know what sex it is?'

'Yes, we know,' said the Greek woman smugly.

After the scan was completed, they called the consultant for his verdict on the results. We had to wait a while. There were only two consultants on duty. 'One of them is a professor. You might get him.' We were told this as if it would be a special treat.

The professor turned up and listened to the reports from his subordinates. He bantered with the men and flirted with the beautiful Greek woman, who seemed to like the attention, while he scanned Kate's stomach again to check their findings.

Then the professor started telling everyone his opinion of the current political situation in the Middle East. He looked at me for a response. I wanted him to concentrate on the baby so I said nothing and turned my head to look at the screen where our baby's brain was waiting to be assessed. He turned to look at the screen as well, but kept moaning about the government. He was a typical male doctor. I saw plenty like him when I was in hospital as a kid. Treated reverentially by patients and junior colleagues, some doctors start to believe they are gods.

While the professor continued his political rant, performing for his sycophantic subordinates, I asked Kate if she still wanted to know the sex of the baby. She did. I was in two minds, but I didn't want to stop her knowing, so I said to the Greek woman, 'Are we right in thinking it's a boy?'

She said, 'If I tell you that, you'll know what sex it is.'

Kate said, 'We've decided we want to know.'

The professor said, 'It's a girl. You're completely wrong.'

I was shocked. 'The reason we thought it was a boy,' I told them, 'was that Kate saw testicles.'

They all laughed smugly. 'That was the umbilical cord,' said the Greek woman.

The professor came to a decision about our baby's brain. 'It's normal,' he said simply.

'Are you sure?' said Kate. 'What's the ventricle measurement?'

He measured it for us. 'Ten millimetres.' He measured it again. This time it was 9 millimetres. 'Normal,' he concluded. He was already leaving the room.

I said to Kate, 'Have you got any questions?' She waved a hand helplessly towards the professor as if to say: what's the point? He was already walking out of the room. Unlike the consultant we saw two weeks ago, this man wasn't giving us much time. 'Thank you,' we said politely to his back and to the other people in the room. Politeness can be a bad habit. This isn't the first time I've left a doctor's office – after being patronised, manipulated, disregarded, misinformed, rushed – and as I've left I've said, 'Thank you.'

We waited in the corridor for our copy of the medical report. Jamal brought it out. He was a nice man, a trainee who hadn't yet acquired the brazen arrogance of his more experienced colleagues. 'You don't have to come for another scan for four weeks,' he said. 'If they were worried, they would say two weeks or one week. Enjoy your pregnancy.'

The important news is that the ventricle size hasn't increased at all. Our baby's brain is officially normal. It feels like we've survived an earthquake. I am relieved, but still suspicious that there are aftershocks to come.

The way they were in the hospital today, abrupt and impatient, makes us think that we'll need to be very clear about our birthing plan if we want to avoid being coerced into doing everything their way. Kate has chosen to have the baby in hospital so that assistance is available if required, but she wants the process of birth to be as natural as possible.

Kate said, 'I wish we didn't know it was a girl now.' We would've been less concerned if it was a boy because of the higher incidence of large ventricles in healthy boys.

There's no point worrying. We must forget about percentages and markers and atrium widths. We must enjoy the pregnancy.

It's a girl ...

Saturday 15 February
An amazing day. We met friends at Charing Cross and joined the march at Trafalgar Square. All motor vehicles were banned from central London. There was a spectacular view along Whitehall where placards bobbed on a river of people. 'MAKE TEA NOT WAR' said one banner. 'FIGHT-ING FOR PEACE IS LIKE SCREWING FOR CHASTITY' said another. 'WAR IS SO 20TH CENTURY' said another. If you believed the police, there were 750,000 people on the march. According to the organisers there were 2 million. Either way it was the largest public demonstration in British history. Similar protests were taking place in 600 cities around the world.

We arrived in Hyde Park in time to hear most of the speeches. One of the speakers referred to the government's attempt to prevent this Stop The War event by claiming that the crowd would destroy the grass in Hyde Park. 'They tried to stop this march on health and safety grounds. We're asking them to stop the war on health and safety grounds.' The sun was setting and my feet were numb. 'It's cold outside but our hearts are warm,' said the American preacher-politician Jesse Jackson. 'It may be winter but all of you together are generating some serious street-heat.' He tried to rouse people into chanting slogans ('Give Peace … A Chance …') but he misjudged the crowd's Englishness and the response was half-hearted and embarrassed. The English will travel hundreds of miles to take part in an anti-war march but don't expect them to chant or sing. He asked everyone to hold hands. Some did, some didn't. Even to prevent a war, the English won't hold hands with strangers.

It was an exhilarating and heartening event. Last week someone asked me if I'm worried about bringing a baby into this world. Today's peaceful worldwide demonstrations, regardless of their political acumen or effectiveness, were a celebration of humanity. I'm happy for our baby to join the party.

Later we went to a fund-raising event on behalf of Cuba. Nine comedians were followed by a dance band. John Hegley recited his poem about Jesus: 'If that's a Good Friday, I wouldn't want a bad one.' We had to leave as the dancing was beginning. The room was too hot and smoky for Kate: 'I was very hot and every time someone lit a cigarette I just felt really angry with them.'

We haven't decided whether to tell friends that our baby is a girl. All day we've had to avoid saying 'she'.

Sunday 16 February   **Week 27**

'We haven't had sex for ages,' said Kate.

'I know.'

'Do you mind?'

'I can't remember. I think I've forgotten how to do it.'

We didn't talk about it any more than that. My desire for sex has diminished in recent weeks. For the first time since … well, for the first time ever. It's ever since Kate started to look like a Weeble. I haven't lost my sexual urges completely. I haven't been turned off. But I'm not exactly turned on either. I'm on standby.

I went to hunt and gather the items on Kate's shopping list, trying not to feel bored. I searched for what Virginia Woolf called 'the sacredness of the ordinary' but I couldn't find it in Sainsbury's.

We have started to call the baby by her name. Kate wanted to look at other names just to make sure that we're not missing something, so we went through a long list of girl's names on a website. We began with French names and moved onto English names, but there was no name we liked more than the one we first thought of.

We've decided that my surname will be the baby's middle name. The baby will have Kate's surname. I don't have a strong attachment to my surname and I quite like the idea of a baby having its mother's surname to counteract hundreds of years of patriarchal lineage. I don't see why the child should have my name after the mother has gone through the agonies of childbirth. Kate wrote the full name for the first time, like a teenager carving a lover's name into a tree.

Kate looked in the bedroom mirror. 'Where's my waist gone?' I didn't have anything useful to say, so I said nothing. Her next question was, 'Has my bum got bigger?' 'No.'

We watched her belly twitch as Alice kicked against it.

Monday 17 February

Over supper we had a Serious Talk about how things are going to work when the baby is here. When and where will I get the private space to work?

Recently I met a writer called Keith who was pessimistic about my hopes of continuing to write after the baby's birth. He knows several writers with babies. He said, 'I'm not saying you have to write off the next five years … but you won't produce your best work.'

It's frustrating. I want to be a good dad, but that's not all I want to be. I'm worried that the prophets of doom are telling the truth and that fatherhood is going to make it impossible to be a writer.

I have moments when I can't remember why I wanted kids. It must've seemed like a good idea at the time. Me Now can't imagine what Me Then was thinking of. We are all at the mercy of other people's decisions: the people we used to be.

If I make an effort, I can guess the reasons why I might have decided I wanted to breed, but I can't actually rekindle the desire itself. Later, the feeling comes back. I recover my optimism and I am able to anticipate the good things.

At the very least, I am fulfilling an important social obligation by providing a taxpayer for the future. Birth rates in England and Wales are at the lowest level since records began. The average woman has 1.64 children over the course of a lifetime – the lowest since 1924. The decrease comes despite multiple births rising by 22 per cent. Women are also leaving it later to start a family; within a decade, the average age has increased from 25.7 years to 27.1 years. Governments are eager for more children. Rampant breeding is their best hope of affording pensions and healthcare for the increasing numbers of elderly people. In Japan, there are more 70-year-olds than 10-year-olds. Björn Borg features in a Swedish poster campaign designed to encourage population growth with the slogan, 'Fuck for the future'.

There are pleasures already. In bed we watched Kate's belly quiver and warp. It has, literally, a life of its own. It's better than watching TV. It trembles and shudders. Tonight the baby was 5.8 on the Richter scale.

Tuesday 18 February
Woke up at 4 am and couldn't get back to sleep. Worrying about all the time slipping away. I waste time thinking about all the time I've wasted already.

For a few weeks, friends have been saying that Kate is blooming, the adjective that only pregnant women are entitled to. Now she feels it as well as looks it. She says that she hasn't been so uncomfortable for the past couple of weeks. Before that, she could feel her muscles straining as her stomach swelled.

We had an antenatal appointment this morning. To get to the hospital we had to walk over the hill. Going uphill, Kate was like a juggernaut in the crawler lane. Going downhill, she was like a runaway train. 'I'm full of energy!' she announced happily as I tried to keep up.

The midwife took blood tests to check iron and blood sugar levels. Then she placed a listening device against Kate's abdomen and, for the first time, we heard our baby's heartbeat. It was 140 beats per minute.

We told the midwife that the baby is a girl. 'Aw, that's nice,' she said. What would she say if it was a boy?

The midwives aren't as knowledgeable as we'd expected. Kate asked if it's safe to wear a maternity belt. A friend has given her one to use later in the pregnancy when she's bigger, but she isn't sure if it's a healthy way to support the bump and reduce the strain on her back. The midwife said, 'Oh yes, I have seen those. I don't know, really.' Kate has read that travel cots are not safe for prolonged use. She asked the midwife why this was. She didn't know. She asked us to let her know if we find out.

I phoned my mum and told her that the baby is a girl. 'Aw, that's nice,' she said. We weren't sure whether to tell her yet because we're afraid that she will immediately rush out and buy armfuls of pink clothing. I dropped several hints that we won't be colour-coding our baby.

Kate was stuck on the sofa again like a beached whale.

Wednesday 19 February

Kate has outgrown her coat.

A hedonistic day, all the sweeter for being stolen. Soon the days will not be my own. They will belong to others.

Terry phoned and invited me to meet him for lunch. I had work to do. And there were still dishes to wash up from last night. 'OK,' I said.

I met Terry outside his workplace and we strolled around St James's Park in the sunshine. He is keen to see Kate while she is big. She has become a freak show.

Walking past a cinema, I noticed that *About Schmidt* was showing at 3.15 pm, so I walked in and bought a ticket, feeling like a free man.

In the evening I met a couple of friends in a pub in Brixton. Anthony and his girlfriend have just bought a three-bedroom house near Peckham Rye for a quarter of a million pounds. He says it needs work doing to it. Well, you can't expect much for a quarter of a million pounds these days. It makes me think we'll never be able to afford to move from our small flat.

Thursday 20 February

Good news. My agent phoned. The good news is that a French theatre director has invited me to attend a ten-day workshop in Normandy. The plan is that we will work on my play with a group of actors and iron out any roughness in the script.

The bad news is that the workshop lasts from 14–23 May. The baby is due on 25 May. I can't go. My play or my baby? No contest. The baby must go on.

But I am pissed off. The baby is already starting to feel like a ball and chain.

My advice to prospective parents is this: when you decide to have kids, write down your reasons because later you might forget what they were, and you'll need to be reminded.

This afternoon on the phone I mentioned my lurking regrets to Kahil, a doting father of three. 'We're having a baby,' I told him. I like saying those words, largely for their shock value. I answered the usual questions. Yes, it was planned. Yes, I am pleased. But I told him that I do occasionally have doubts. He said, 'We all do, but once it's there … I heard someone talking about the settlements in the West Bank, saying they are facts on the ground. That's what babies are. They're facts on the ground.' And we just have to get on with it.

This evening I phoned Nana and told her that it's a girl. 'Aw, that's lovely,' she said.

I also spoke to one of my aunties and thanked her for a Christmas present. A mother of two boys, she assured me that having children is worthwhile even though 'it's hard work, it's no good saying it's not' and 'your life's not your own'.

Friday 21 February

The truth is, if there was a button I could press to return our lives to a pre-pregnancy state, I wouldn't press it. Walking up mountains, writing plays, having babies – anything worth doing in life involves moments of doubt and difficulty. The main struggle is against yourself.

It was a lovely sunny morning next to the Thames. I was waiting to meet a couple of friends. It was low tide and the river was in one of its languid moods. I sat on the wall forming the South Bank, my legs dangling over the shingle. In the distance, Tower Bridge looked like an enchanted castle in the hazy sunshine.

It was near here, on a wooden pier in front of the OXO Tower, that I first kissed Kate. After eating in a Japanese restaurant, we had ended up strolling along the river. I wasn't sure how much she liked me, but I decided to take the risk. It was the first time I'd ever kissed someone without knowing that the odds of success were in my favour. Out of shyness and cowardice, I had spent all the previous years of my life only kissing women who'd make it obvious that they were interested.

The pier was cosy in the late evening darkness. A galaxy of streetlights twinkled on the Thames. St Paul's Cathedral floated on the city like a ghostly ocean liner. It seemed like a conducive moment. When I leant over and kissed her, her mouth was hard and closed. It was like kissing a block of wood. Later, as we said goodnight next to Westminster Bridge, she kissed me with more enthusiasm, having got used to the idea. Now it was my turn to be unresponsive. I kissed her back politely but not passionately, uncertain of her feelings and my own. It wasn't until the next weekend, lying in the long grass on Hampstead Heath with a sprawling view of London that we hardly looked at, that we kissed each other properly.

When my friends turned up, we crossed the river and on the steps of St Paul's Cathedral we joined a small group of people for a walking tour of the City of London. Today is a day of free guided tours given by the Blue Badge tour guides. Our guide was a former actor who had played Toad in the theatre version of *The Wind in the Willows*. Toad took us through the local streets named after the tradesmen who used to work there. Bread Street (bakers), Milk Street (dairymen) and Friday Street (fishmongers). We passed several of Wren's churches including one whose circular altar, designed by Henry Moore, is a beautiful white slab of stone nicknamed The Camembert. Each street contained remnants of the city's Roman, Elizabethan and Victorian past. Behind the Bank of England, Toad pointed out the Church of St Margaret of Lothbury, the patron saint of childbirth.

Birth preserves the dying art of talking to strangers. When they find out that you're having a baby, other parents willingly offer their own celebratory or consolatory stories. This afternoon I had an appointment with the osteopath, Beverley, and I told her about our recent scare with the scan results. She said that she was given a big fright in the eighth month of her second pregnancy when the midwives measured her belly and sent her for another ultrasound scan. After the scan she was told that the foetus was too small for this stage of pregnancy. The too-small foetus is now a perfectly healthy little boy (but not too little).

Kate's friend was told she had a one-in-three chance of having a baby with Down's syndrome. The baby was born without any abnormalities of any kind.

The more I read and hear, the more I realise that almost every pregnancy and birth has a complication that scares the parents.

Some of her friends at work keep telling Kate how small she is. They mean well. They're trying to say, kindly, that she isn't fat. But she wants to be big. She wants to be undeniably, demonstrably pregnant. I told her not to worry. It's hard to reassure someone simultaneously that she is big but not fat.

We spent five minutes assessing her ankles, trying to decide if they're swollen or not. They are.

Saturday 22 February

An antenatal appointment in the hospital. When Kate's name was called, I stayed in the waiting room reading my book. A man and a woman examined Kate's belly, applying gel painfully and prodding her roughly with medical implements. Kate called my name and I came into the room. I explained to her that I thought she'd wanted me to stay in the waiting room. I watched as the examination continued. The procedure seemed unnecessarily violent. They were hurting Kate but I felt unable to intervene, so she just had to lie there and suffer.

That was Kate's dream last night.

'I felt so powerless.'

'I promise you I won't just sit there and read,' I said.

Friends came round for dinner. Afterwards we went to see Chekhov's *Three Sisters* in a theatre behind Dulwich College, an ambitious choice for an amateur dramatic company. It was more amateur than dramatic. The greatest moments of suspense were provided by the 80-year-old woman playing the nurse. Whenever she began a sentence, you never knew if she would remember the end of it. There were long pauses while she waited for someone to say the next line, until she realised that the next line was hers.

One of our friends gave us a lift home in his Porsche. I wedged myself into the back seat. I had to sit sideways with my head squashed under the sloping rear window. Feeling claustrophobic, I was glad when the journey was over. It took me five minutes to get out of the car. I had to fold my legs at strange angles and resort to several yoga positions. It was like trying to get out of a washing machine.

We said thank you and goodnight to our friend. As we crossed the road in front of our house, we heard the repeated honking of a car horn. I turned and saw a car speeding towards us. The speed limit on this residential street is 30mph but this idiot was travelling at 50mph at least. I waved my arm up and down to suggest that the driver should slow down, but he kept accelerating. He clearly objected to the sight of pedestrians on his racetrack.

Then I saw that Kate was lying on the road. In a hurry to get out of the way of this madman, she had stumbled and twisted her ankle. Luckily she had fallen between two parked cars. The car sped past.

Kate wasn't hurt. I phoned the police and gave them the registration number. (We heard nothing more about it.)

Sunday 23 February   Week 28

A day at the seaside. We came here nearly four years ago for our first date. On that occasion we took our bikes on the train to Brighton, cycled eastwards between the cliffs and the sea, then pedalled on to the South Downs. Her hesitation when we'd first kissed in London made me think that she wanted to take things slowly. Then, in a field of buttercups and cows, she proved me wrong.

Today we left our bikes at home. Engineering works meant that the train from Victoria to Brighton was diverted and took an extra hour. I was pleased. I love these old trains with their slamming doors and shaking windows. Instead of air conditioning, they have air. We had one of the small carriages to ourselves so Kate was able to lie down across the seats and snooze as we trundled through the sunshine past Arundel Castle.

We got off the train in Hove where we met her brother, Phil. He drove us to a football pitch in Shoreham-by-Sea at the foot of the South Downs. We were just in time for the kick-off. The goalkeeper for Hove Park Colts Under-11s was Kate's brother's wife's sister's little boy. I cheered him on as if he was my own flesh and blood, although I was advised that spectators are not encouraged to get too excited ever since an over-involved parent bit off a piece of a referee's ear. Today's match passed without violent incident. Ryan played well and his team won 1–0.

For lunch we went to Donatello's, a pizza restaurant in Brighton, and occupied a table for nine. Four adults and five kids aged 13, 10, 7, 3 and 1. Plus two unborn infants. Since I last saw her, Holly, the three-year-old, has learnt how to drink from a glass. She has also learnt how to turn it upside down, spilling the contents all over the table. She did this twice. Chloe said to me with heavy irony, 'Are you looking forward to having kids?'

Her sister, Linda, a mother of four, warned me to be prepared for biting and swearing during the labour.

Later, Ryan and I stood at the edge of the sea and skimmed stones across its surface. We were surprised by a big wave, which rushed up the shingle and soaked our shoes and socks.

They're all nice kids. Sweet-natured and fun to be with. A day with children hasn't put me off parenthood. I am looking forward to it slightly more, actually. Participation is better than anticipation. The problem with pregnancy, this liminal state between childlessness and parenthood, is that what you're going to lose is more conspicuous than what you're going to gain.

Back in London, I said, 'Alice will be here soon.' We keep realising this, forgetting it, then realising it again. 'It's only three months!' said Kate. Three months! And then we'll be expected to know what to do.

Monday 24 February

I went to Guy's Hospital this morning for some tests. Doctors are research-ing the prevalence of asthma and allergies among the population of South London and I got a letter inviting me to be one of the study sample. A bespectacled man with bushy eyebrows and a bushy moustache – the twin brother of Groucho Marx – measured my lung capacity and put droplets on my skin, containing the essence of dust, dogs and cats, to see if I came out in a rash. I think I was a disappointment to him. Everything was nor-mal. The final procedure was a blood test. Groucho Marx said to me, 'I'll have to ask you to lie down since you're a man.'

'Why?'

'We've found that men tend to feel more queasy.'

'Why?'

'I think it's because women have been through more. Like childbirth.'

I felt slighted. I've had dozens of blood tests without buckling at the knees. I lay on the couch and managed not to pass out despite being a member of the weaker sex.

Kate woke up screaming during the night. 'ARRRGGGGHHHHH!' I snapped awake. She was holding her leg. 'CRAMP!' she said. 'ARRRRRGGGGGGHHH!' It was a full-throated roar as if someone had stabbed her with a carving knife or an elephant had trodden on her foot. I said, perhaps unkindly, 'If you're like this about cramp, what are you going to be like during childbirth?' After a while, the pain went away and she was able to go back to sleep.

Her screams were disturbing. It made me realise that I am going to have to watch her go through terrible pain, possibly for hours. It will be like watching her being tortured, and there won't be much I can do to help. I don't believe that rubbing scented oils into her back is going to make the pain go away.

Tuesday 25 February

Mamie, Kate's French grandmother, has broken her leg. Her femur snapped when she got out of bed. Kate asked me to take some photos of the bump to send to France.

We may or may not be in the third trimester already. One book says it begins in week 27, another book says week 29. I was pleased to see that 'at 28 weeks the baby is said to be viable'. In other words, it is considered to have a good chance of survival if born. The baby weighs about 2½ pounds, and will probably double in weight before she is born.

We're reading the pregnancy books again. Now that we can again believe that our baby is healthy and the pregnancy is normal, the books seem relevant to us.

We know that the baby is heavier. Kate is noticing the extra weight when she tries to stand up.

She keeps scratching her belly. Her skin itches as it stretches.

Wednesday 26 February

Kate was standing naked in front of the mirror admiring her bump. 'It's beautiful, isn't it?' 'It is.' It is.

I went to see a play called *The Green Man* at the Bush Theatre with my agent, Laura. She is remarkably optimistic about the effects of parenthood on writers. Several of her clients have children and she reckons that you write nothing for the first three months after the birth and then things get back to normal and roll along. She speaks with the unequivocal confidence of someone who hasn't got any kids of her own.

Thursday 27 February

I've arranged travel insurance for our holiday. The insurance company won't insure pregnant women after 28 weeks so the policy doesn't cover anything relating to the pregnancy. We can be insured for abseiling or hang-gliding but not for pregnancy.

There are constant unsolicited reminders that birth is a near-death experience. I turned on the radio and heard that four babies die every day because of medical errors. Thirty mothers die every year as a result of avoidable medical mistakes. England is at the bottom of the European league table when it comes to preventable deaths in childbirth. It says that avoidable mistakes account for 53 per cent of baby deaths during labour and the first six weeks of life. That's 800 babies over a five year period.

Pregnancy is forcing me to confront my attitude to disability. For all parents there's a risk – small but actual – that their baby could be born with a physical or mental impairment. We have decided to take the consequences of that risk. Part of me feels ashamed that part of me dreads the prospect of having to care for a severely disabled child. I've had limited contact with disabled people. And they are excluded from the media unless they've accomplished something exceptional. You can get the impression that disabled people are all Olympic athletes, spending their days competing in wheelchair marathons and playing wheelchair basketball. Today I was flipping through an old magazine and came across a touching and inspiring interview with the former Formula 1 racing driver Damon Hill. He was just starting out as a driver when his first child, Ollie, was born with Down's syndrome. 'It was a shock. But with children, there's only one kind of resolution. You just accept them, do what you can for them and love them … All I can say is that Ollie's just a wonderful human being and I learn as much from him as I do from my other children, so we consider ourselves lucky.'

Kate has a new toy. Her bra. Without preamble she lifted her jumper and exposed two white hammocks supporting her giant breasts. It's for breastfeeding. With a click she unhooked one of the hammocks and peeled it away, exposing a dark nipple. Then she repeated the trick on the other side. She has wanted to do this all day. She wanted to show her friends at work, but wisely decided it would be inappropriate.

Often we sit in front of the telly, watching the ten o'clock news, and I fiddle with her hair in the way she likes. She has complained that I'm not giving her enough massages.

'You get a head massage every night,' I pointed out.

'But I got that before I was pregnant.'

Tonight, when I didn't respond immediately to her demand for a back massage, she said: 'You're supposed to be mollycoddling me.' I asked if she had any other complaints. She did. We have run out of mineral water.

Friday 28 February

I went to Sainsbury's and bought 9 litres of mineral water.

Kate phoned from a bus between Kennington and Brixton. 'Alice is kicking lots.'

When she got home, she announced: 'I don't think I've had a pooh for three days.'

I phoned Sarah. I called at the wrong time. But there's never a right time to call someone who has three children. Two of her children had friends visiting. Sarah was just preparing food for seven little people with big appetites, so our conversation was very short. We agreed to talk another time. I will have to get used to this. Deferring conversations, deferring friendships, deferring the rest of life.

Kate dropped a piece of paper on the floor and had to ask me to pick it up for her. The bump is starting to get in the way. She is finding it difficult to bend forward. She has to eat with outstretched arms. Every meal requires the balance and coordination skills of an egg-and-spoon race.

Sleeping is another thing that can't be taken for granted any more. She is struggling to get comfortable at night. 'Just for the last two or three nights, I'm getting little pains in my joints.'

I stayed up late. When I went to bed, I found a large pillow in my place. It was propped against her back to stop her lying in the wrong position. She has read that certain sleeping positions can squash the placenta and reduce the baby's oxygen supply. Getting into bed is like an obstacle course.

Saturday 1 March

I found Kate climbing a ladder into the loft, looking for her sandals. She likes doing things herself.

'You shouldn't be climbing ladders.'

'It's OK.'

I can't really afford this holiday. But life is short. And when it isn't short, it's cruel. Kate phoned Mamie. She has been staying in a convalescence home near Toulouse since breaking her leg. She sounded troubled. She said that she had done a pooh some time ago and she was still waiting for a nurse to take it away.

It's a joyful feeling, setting off with a rucksack on your back, even one this heavy. I am carrying her stuff as well as mine.

Kate was tired. The area of her body between her bump and her breasts – quite a narrow valley now – felt tight, constricted. At the airport lounge she lay on the seats with her legs raised. 'Why am I so tired? I hope I haven't ended my energetic period just as we're going to Rome.'

On the plane, she asked for two cups of hot water into which she dipped a dandelion leaf tea bag. Dandelion is supposed to alleviate swelling. Pregnant women can turn into balloon animals on an aeroplane. Kaz Cooke writes that 'planes always make my feet swell up, but now it seems to work on my whole body … have gone quite bullfroggy around the face'. Kate was spared this.

In front of us was an empty row of three seats. Kate stood up to move there for the extra space. The stewardess told her sternly that the seat belt signs were illuminated because of turbulence, but when she noticed that Kate was pregnant, allowed her to move anyway. But she warned her to be careful 'because you're not insured'. Kate safely completed the 2-yard journey.

After a bus ride from the airport, we took a metro to Policlinico. When we walked into our hotel room, Kate said: 'It's like a cell.' The room is lit by two 24-inch tubular bulbs on the ceiling. The walls are stark white. When we turn the lights on, the effect is blinding, like an atomic explosion.

The floor consists of hard, cold, mottled tiles. There is no chair. There is nothing soft in the room. Even the bed sheets are thin and crispy. The towels are the size and thickness of napkins.

The toilet and shower are along the hall. Kate went first. When she came back, she said: 'It's a good thing you brought loo roll.'

Inside the vast, ugly green wardrobe, the clothes rail is about eight feet off the floor; we have to stand on tiptoe to hang up our clothes.

Kate swapped the pillows so that I got the lumpy one.

For this we are paying €45 (£35) per night. I feel ashamed that I can't afford something plusher for my pregnant beloved. I suggested that we can look for somewhere better tomorrow, but she insisted that this is fine.

Our guidebook says this hotel used to be a convent. I suspect the nuns moved out because it was too uncomfortable.

Sunday 2 March   Week 29

After a draughty night, we opened the shutters and found cool grey skies and heavy rain.

'Heaven!' said Kate when we walked into a pasticceria for breakfast. We stood at the counter and warmed ourselves with croissants and thick hot chocolate. People seemed to have dressed up for breakfast. A man in a yellow waistcoat. A man in a leather jacket, defiantly wearing sunglasses even though he was indoors on a grey day. We ordered two more croissants. 'This is heaven,' repeated Kate.

We strolled around the perimeter of the Colosseum, a dramatic sight under low black clouds. Gladiators were poking nervous Japanese tourists with plastic swords. Other gladiators were talking on mobile phones and wearing Gucci sunglasses (which they hid behind their backs when posing for photos with the tourists).

The Colosseum has inspired painters and poets, but Kate wasn't so impressed. She said, 'There should be places for pregnant women to lie on their back with their legs up.'

We met her Italian friend Giulia whose flat has a vast balcony with a view across the city to St Peter's Cathedral and the sculptural trees on the Aventine Hill.

Kate crosses the Roman roads like a frightened, bedazzled rabbit. Giulia has a more defiant technique, striding boldly in front of the traffic, glaring at speeding drivers and daring them not to stop.

In Italy it costs less to stand at the bar than to sit at a table. Kate said, 'I can't do standing still. My legs start to tingle.' So we sat. Sitting down costs a minimum of €5 unless it's in a church.

When we stopped to rest in the Santa Maria della Consolazione, she propped her legs on the back of the pew in front. The verger, who was changing candles, glared at her. But God didn't seem to mind. We weren't struck by lightning.

Rome forces you to walk. Every street is an array of pleasures. Something amazing, another marvellous building or piazza, is always around the corner. So we kept walking a little bit further.

We ate in a popular restaurant, Il Brillo Parlante. Kate was temporarily trapped in the toilets because she was too wide to squeeze past the other women in there.

We watched a film, *Chicago*, at Piazza della Repubblica. We emerged from the cinema at midnight. The gates to the metro station were locked. Taxis were few and full. We walked home in the drizzle. Kate had to sit on a wall at the roadside. She said, 'I think I've done too much today.'

And so to bed. I asked, 'What was the thing you liked most today?'

She said, 'Lying here right now.'

Monday 3 March

The state of one's bowels, always a concern for travellers, becomes the focal point of existence when one of you is pregnant. Kate has been constipated for a while. Now she has diarrhoea. I woke up in the night as she was getting back into bed after a prolonged visit to the toilet along the hall. She gave me a vivid description. 'All liquid and bubbling. Long farts.'

She was scared that the baby was coming because she felt it moving lower as we walked yesterday and she has read that diarrhoea is a sign that you're about to give birth.

It was cold enough for the Romans to be wearing scarves. We strolled around the Spanish Steps then ate two plates of spaghetti in the café famous for its ice cream, Giolitti. In cool weather, some locals have mastered the art of making a coffee last for half a day. Two Italian men abandoned their table, leaving a mountain of fag ends in the ashtray. One waiter complained to another, 'From eight o'clock this morning they just had a cappuccino!'

As we walked through Piazza Navona, the sun came out. We saw a glamorous woman with coiffured hair, bold red lipstick and deep black mascara. She looked, if not like a film star, at least like a popular actress in a daytime soap. But she was pulling a trolley with a bin on it. She was a refuse collector. Italy's refuse collectors dress as if they're strolling along a catwalk.

We bought slices of pizza and wandered past the Fontana di Trevi. When you're pregnant, it's important never to be too far away from food. Rome becomes a giant buffet. Kate is trying not to drink wine or coffee. In Italy this is a form of torture.

At the hotel Kate asked, now that she's pregnant, 'Do you not find me as attractive?'

I said, 'Of course I do.'

We started to make love. Initially I was reluctant because it felt like there were three of us in the bed. But I overcame those reservations fairly quickly. But she felt fragile 'down there', so we gave up. My feelings, briefly awakened, went back to sleep again. I'm relieved, at least, that my libido seems to be dormant rather than dead.

Tuesday 4 March

Kate is restless in bed now. It's like sleeping with an egg whisk. I woke up in the night to find her trying to push me away with her forearm. She said, confusingly, 'But I like it when you snuggle up to me.' My job, apparently, is to put my arm around her when she's cold and to move to the far side of the bed when she wants more space. I must detect these desires and execute these manoeuvres instantly in my sleep. It's that simple.

She can't get the towel around her waist when she goes to the shower.

She says that she is grumpier, less patient than she used to be. I said that she isn't so grumpy. By the end of the day, I had changed my mind.

All Rome leads to roads. Sooner or later, you'll have to cross one of them. Given the choice of crossing a road with a pregnant woman or a frightened rabbit, I would choose the rabbit every time for its superior road sense.

The traffic lights changed when we were halfway across a busy main road. Kate froze on the spot. I kept going, because the cars were waiting for us, and took her elbow to usher her (as I saw it) to safety. She accused me of pushing her into the traffic. The debate continued for some time. She had the final word. The final word was 'off'.

'Silly girl.'

'Fuck off.'

She gets easily irritated. Not just by me. By the rude member of staff in the Vatican who seemed to think he was God rather than one of His employees. By the member of staff in the metro station who didn't have a map of Rome's transport system (nobody does).

Rome, as every pregnant woman knows, is built on seven hills. Hands on her waist, I pushed her up one of them. So much for taking things easier. We walked miles again.

In the grounds of the Villa Borghese, we hired a bike, a side-by-side tandem. It seemed like a good idea at the time. It was a heavy metal trolley. Confronted by the slightest incline, I had to get out and push. If I overtook other tandems, or went over the tiniest bump in the path, she rebuked me for reckless driving.

Under the shade of the trees, we came across an International Chocolate Exhibition. Several hundred stalls were selling chocolate from every region of Italy. For me it was paradise. For Kate it was another circle of hell. Chocolate aggravates heartburn so she had to resist the chocolate spoons and chocolate spanners, chocolate pasta, chocolate jigsaws, chocolate with chilli, chocolate of every shape and hue. I, on the other hand, walked past every stall, dawdling at the ones with free samples.

There's nothing like a dome. Inside St Peter's Cathedral, we took the elevator as high as it would go. Then we had to climb 320 ever-narrowing steps to the top of the dome. Kate wanted to pause for a rest along the way. 'Spaghetti?' said an Italian man cheekily as he overtook us, suggesting that Kate's bump and fatigue were the result of overeating. A minute later, we passed him and his partner as they rested on the stairs. 'Ravioli?' I asked.

After climbing to the top of St Peter's Cathedral, Kate felt like a siesta. We hopped on a bus without knowing where it was going. It was heading in completely the wrong direction. We stayed aboard anyway because it was warm and Kate wanted to sit down with her legs resting on the seat opposite.

Eventually we found our way to a restaurant near Piazza Navona. Then we meandered through cobbled streets and collected a small ice cream on the way. Even the small ice creams are huge.

'Alice isn't moving very much. But maybe that's because I'm walking around a lot and can't feel it.'

'I'm sure it is.'

Wednesday 5 March

We are in Rome. One of the world's most beautiful cities. She said, 'I'm worried that when I'm tightening my pelvic floor muscles, I'm tightening my anal muscles and that's stopping me poohing.'

'It's fine, lovey.'

'That's your response to everything. When I'm in labour you'll be saying "It's fine, it's fine." And then you *will* get a slap.'

We went to the Vatican. There was airport-style security, but the man with the metal detector let Kate through without scanning her.

Every Wednesday the frail Pope meets the public. Eight thousand people in one room. He was wheeled on to stage on a trolley. As he entered, he raised a shaky hand off the railing and waved. The crowd applauded rapturously. He slumped in a chair and blessed everyone in eight languages, his voice slurring with age and illness. After the speeches and blessings, which lasted for over an hour, he was wheeled off the stage. Resting his bum against the railing on the trolley, he risked waving with both hands at the same time. It was a showman's finale. The crowd clapped and cheered and whistled.

Another day of sun and blue skies. We bought giant portions of pizza and sat among the market stalls in the Campo de' Fiori. We walked to the Forum. By dusk we had arrived in the old square in Trastevere.

The cheerful lawlessness of Italian road-users is less endearing when you're pregnant. We've seen numerous cars and scooters going through red lights. In Trastevere a man on a scooter nearly ran us over because he was busy writing a text message as he rode along the pavement. His brakes brought him to a halt inches in front of us. He looked apologetic.

I'm spending a lot of time wondering what I've done wrong. What crime have I committed to make her mood so sour? She admits that she is 'irritated and ill-humoured'. Glum-faced, she blames it on her constipation.

She spent 15 minutes on the loo and returned with a disappointed sigh. 'I didn't manage anything.'

The Pope has blessed our baby but really we need him to bless her bowels.

Thursday 6 March

On the metro, someone stood up to give Kate a seat. But an old man sat down before she could get there. So a woman gave up her seat instead. It was like a strange dance.

We went to the train station to enquire about tickets to Florence and Siena. Kate went to the loo. 'I managed a pellet about that big.' Her fingers made a circle about the size of a pea. The first thing she has produced in three days.

Ostia Antica is an abandoned Roman town, half an hour by train from Rome. We walked along an ancient cobbled road, trying not to step on geckos and giant pine cones. The pine trees had tall trunks with a globe of greenery at the summit, neat and pert, as if they'd just been to the hairdresser's for a perm. We spent six hours walking around the ruins, and could've happily stayed longer. The beautiful amphitheatre, dating from the Augustan era, used to entertain audiences of 3,500 people. Today there were about 50 tourists, sunbathing. We found a Roman bakery whose circular millstone used to be pushed by donkeys that were blindfolded to stop them becoming dizzy. There were three-storey Roman houses, grand civic buildings, mosaics and wall paintings. Ostia Antica makes Stonehenge look like a bunch of pebbles. We sat among the ruins of a building and ate a picnic.

I went to use the toilets in the visitors' building. When I emerged, Kate said accusingly, 'Did you pooh?'

I admitted that I had poohed.

'It's not fair.'

I tried to think of something consoling to say about constipation. 'It's normal, lovey. It's fine.'

The last time I said something was fine she tongue-lashed me. So I wasn't sure what her reaction would be now. 'Thank you,' she said, and gave me a kiss.

Beyond the Capitolium, behind the Forum, we found the ornate Latrines.

'So they all came here to shit. The bastards.'

'Why are they bastards?'

'Because they could shit.'

Back in Rome, she decided to buy a laxative, checking with the chemist that it was safe for pregnant women. It made her feel sick.

Kate is receiving random goodwill from strangers. 'Good luck!' said a woman at the Vatican. *'Auguri!'* said a man on the metro. Tonight we went to see a play. During the interval, the woman serving drinks behind the bar allowed Kate to take a drink into the auditorium because 'the baby will be hungry'.

Friday 7 March

'I managed a little pooh,' said Kate. 'About that big.' She made a circle with her fingers, about the size of a marble.

We spent a couple of hours exploring the Colosseum. When we emerged, the toilets had just closed. A large crowd was being turned away. But the female toilet attendant allowed Kate to use the facilities because she was pregnant.

Unfortunately this privilege wasn't extended to pregnant men.

The attendant said to Kate, 'I remember when I was pregnant. All the toilets were mine.' (*Tutti i bagni erano i miei.*) It was a colossal success. Kate reported that she had produced a golf ball.

We took the metro to Piazza di Spagna. Increasingly tired and grumpy, and failing to find pizza, we went to Giolitti for an emergency transfusion of ice cream. She complained to the staff because a waiter failed to appear within 60 seconds.

At Piazza Barberini, an internet café called Easy Everything turned out to be one of the highlights of the holiday for Kate. 'I had another pooh,' she reported. 'The biggest one yet.'

Near Piazza Navona we found a restaurant recommended by the guidebook and settled into our seats for an evening of whining and dining. The menu was almost entirely seafood, which pregnant women are told to avoid because of the risk of listeria. And people were smoking. Kate was too tired to make conversation. I found myself restless, frustrated, thinking that a pregnant woman is a slow dopey lump.

We eavesdropped on the conversation at the next table. A middle-aged man, a university professor, was dining with a young female student. When the student went to the toilet, the professor asked the young waitress if she'd like to have dinner with him sometime.

I don't think we should teach Alice to speak Italian. I don't want to make it easier for Italian men to communicate with her.

Kate was tetchy, irritated by the smoke and the slow service. She grumbled because the waiter was late bringing the bill.

The buses are unpredictable. Eventually one turned up, heading in the right direction. On board, she was pensive. I took a risk and asked her the question. 'What are you thinking about?'

She said that she is more irritable than usual and impatient if she doesn't get what she wants straight away. Like not getting the food she craved in the restaurant. And she is more tearful. She says the last time she remembers feeling this frustrated was when she was three years old.

'I wish you'd told me earlier,' I said. 'When you're like this, I feel like I'm failing in some way. It helps to know it isn't always my fault.'

Normally the most equable of people, her levels of tetchiness and irritability are almost on a level with mine now. If my internal organs were being slowly displaced and squashed, I'd be grumpy too.

Saturday 8 March
Kate feels as if her trousers are too tight, but they're not. It's her skin that's tight.

We took the 9.03 from Rome to Florence. We had booked a Eurostar train rather than an Intercity. It cost twice as much but it meant an hour less of comfortless sitting for Kate. We were sitting in a non-smoking carriage but she could smell smoke. It came from a man sitting two seats behind us; he wasn't smoking, but the stench exuded from him.

We spent the day wandering around Florence with an old friend, James, and his girlfriend Paola. After a long lunch, we took a bus up the hill to admire the panoramic view from Piazzale Michelangelo. Then a long walk down the hill took us across the famous bridge, the Ponte Vecchio. Ice cream in Florence is half the size and twice the price as Rome. Kate ate three scoops and then complained that she was cold. So we all sat in a café near the train station.

James asked what we're going to call our child. I told him it's a secret. So he tried to guess. He has a theory that parents give their kids names beginning with their own initial. (His mum is called Joyce.) So he started to guess girl's names beginning with A and B. I managed to distract him before he got to Alice.

James's appearance and outlook haven't changed much over the years. He is 39 but looks about 25. He has written two songs that recently appeared in the Italian pop charts (the second one got as high as number 27). He presents a programme on a television station in Parma, teaching English to Italian children. I sensed that his girlfriend wanted me to promote the idea of parenthood and settling down, but James is adamant that he doesn't want kids. He says he is a child inside. 'Having children isn't a duty.'

They caught a train back to Parma. We boarded a train to Siena.

'Why do *we* want kids?' asked Kate.

'Remind me,' I said.

'I've forgotten.' But she tried to remember. 'The biological clock was a big factor. And also … it's another journey, another holiday.'

'A holiday?'

'Our holidays aren't always easy or relaxing. They're something we do together.'

Parenthood as a long holiday is an appealing notion. That's called looking on the bright side.

She asked me why I wanted children.

I said that the clock is a factor. Not only her biological clock, but also my psychological clock: an awareness that years are passing and that, if we're ever going to have children, we may as well have them fairly soon. At 37, I'm relatively old to become a dad. But I have a reasonable chance of living long enough to see my children become adults. It's an adventure and it's a risk. We're taking the risk that the adventure of having kids is worthwhile.

I asked if she's sure that she wants kids. She said that she is sure, but she does have moments when she has … not doubts … but uncertainties about the effects it will have. On her career. On our relationship. She thinks it might make me think she is just 'a stupid mum', bovine and mumsy. She worries about not being a good enough mum.

I like the idea that the baby is something we're doing together. Sometimes the baby feels like something that's being done to us. I mustn't forget that I volunteered for this, whatever it is.

The taxi ride from the station, through Siena's narrow undulating streets, between high stone buildings, was like riding the rapids through a canyon. Our hotel room has luxury amenities including chairs, a bin, a bedside lamp and a view of the Piazza Indipendenza. Best of all, from the point of view of a pregnant woman, it has an en suite bathroom. 'This is heaven!' said Kate as she got into a bed with clean sheets for the first time in a week.

Kate has been to Siena before. She wanted to take me to the *Campo*, the medieval square. We left the hotel, walked around a couple of corners and there it was, floodlit and magnificent. In a bar we ate panini and admired cakes as monumental and magnificent as the buildings. Another marvellous day in Italy.

Sunday 9 March   Week 30

In the morning, sunlight and church bells seeped through the shutters.

Not long after breakfast, Kate was hungry again. So only a brief stroll separated breakfast from lunch, and along the way we discussed where to go for supper. Italy is one long meal.

She looks at her reflection in shop windows, trying to see her bottom.

Walking across the Piazza della Libertà, Kate suddenly screamed. 'Aaaah! Alice! You're squashing my bladder. I nearly peed myself.'

Siena's rolling streets exhausted Kate. She sat on the brick floor of the scallop-shaped *campo*, which is described by the *Rough Guide* as the finest piazza in Italy, and revived herself with an ice cream. Back in the hotel, we lay on the bed for five minutes and woke up an hour later. Then it was time to eat again.

There's an old saying: 'In France, the food makes you appreciate the genius of the chef. In Italy, the food makes you appreciate the genius of God.'

Monday 10 March

We had sex this morning. We were slightly distracted, wondering what the baby was making of it all.

Then the day got even better. She emerged from the toilet with a smile. 'I poohed!'

We went by bus to San Gimignano. From a distance, it looks like a city of skyscrapers perched on a Tuscan hill. A cluster of medieval towers have made it famous as a 'Medieval Manhattan' and the resemblance to an American city is increased when you discover that the streets are full of Americans.

A short walk was followed by pizza. Another short walk was followed by ice cream. An ice cream here is big enough for two people, but Kate is two people, so we got one each.

It's only a small town but the local pensioners, sitting on a wall in the sunshine, had plenty to say to each other. Elderly Italians gossiped and young American women wrote their journals. We sat on a wall watching the view, and watching tourists watching the view.

Away from the tourists and trinket shops, we ambled along the narrow path outside the old town walls, riding a roller coaster of hills, and felt glad that we had made the effort to travel. In the rose-tinted glow of a Tuscan twilight we allowed ourselves to hope that travelling with kids will be possible.

The sun set while we waited at the bus stop. The bus arrived and climbed a hill. The sun reappeared. As the bus rose and dipped on the twisting, undulating road, we were treated to 15 sunsets.

On the bus she felt stiff around her chest. Below the bump is a muscle, she says, that feels as though it might snap and everything will spill out of her.

When he found out that Kate spoke Italian, the bus driver appointed himself our tour guide and pointed out a fortified village on a hilltop. He asked us where we're from. London? He has never been there. We told him that we're on a last holiday before we have our first child.

The old woman sitting behind us said, 'You can't travel when you have kids. My husband travelled all over, but when we got married, I told him to forget about travelling.'

'You missed out,' the bus driver told her.

'I know I missed out, I missed a lot!' said the old woman, laughing. 'But you can't travel with kids. There's too much to worry about.'

'You can travel,' insisted the bus driver. 'You just have to not worry. If you start worrying, you never stop.'

'Have you travelled much?' I asked him.

'No,' he admitted.

'Why not?'

He shrugged. 'I have two kids.'

Back in Siena, we found a restaurant not far from the cinema. We walked in and almost walked out again. A man was smoking a pipe next to the only available table. I explained to the waiter that we didn't want to smoke, and gestured to Kate's stomach. The man with the pipe overheard.

'I will not smoke any more,' he said in English.

It was an unconventional restaurant. The waiter sat on a chair at our table as he noted down our order. The chef/owner appeared from the kitchen and asked all his customers not to smoke because there was a pregnant woman in the room. We thanked everyone as we left. '*Auguri!*' they all chorused.

I pushed Kate up a hill to the tiny, cold cinema converted from a fresco-lined church. We watched Charlie Chaplin speaking Italian in *Il Grande*

Dittatore. The screen was a white rectangle erected in front of a marble fresco. Ancient paintings adorned the walls. The film finished half an hour after midnight. Kate fell asleep a couple of times. Alice was kicking a lot during the film. Which cheered Kate up, because she was worried that she hadn't felt any movements all day.

Kate huffs and puffs when walking up slopes and even when she's putting on her shoes in a morning.

Tuesday 11 March

Our last day. We munched pizza while lying on the *campo* in the sunshine. I got pigeon shit on my jacket. Then I climbed up Siena's famous Mangia tower. Despite conquering the hills of Rome and Tuscany this week, Kate felt that the tower, with 400 steps, was beyond her capabilities. She stayed at ground level, looking at shoes and fruit.

It was the right decision. Apart from the physical challenge, she would have been too wide. Inside the narrow staircase, I felt claustrophobic as the brick walls scraped my hips.

We headed back to Rome. The local train from Siena was full of school kids. It was hard to ignore the two teenagers near us, a pretty girl and a spotty lad, who were snogging passionately, lips clamped together. Every movement was slow and intense. Kate stared at them, worried that they couldn't breathe. They were oblivious with lust, uninterested in the scenery. We could've had sex ourselves and they wouldn't have noticed. After half an hour, the girl got off the train; the boy stayed on and started doing his algebra homework. He'd already done his biology.

'We've had good snogs in our day,' said Kate.

'Are our days over?'

So we snogged, to prove that we still could. But we were laughing too much; and Kate couldn't breathe; and the seats were uncomfortable.

We arrived in Rome at 5.20 pm or so. Our flight was due to leave Ciampino at 8.45 pm. We should've gone straight to the airport. Instead we wanted to snatch a last hour in Rome. We took a packed metro to Flaminio and joined the *passeggiata* along Via del Corso. We reached the Spanish Steps in time for sunset, watching all the colours in the sky behind St Peter's Cathedral, and ate a final ice cream.

We arrived at the airport only half an hour before our flight was due to leave.

Kate jumped off the bus and ran across the concourse. I shouted at her to stop running. We were flustered, hassled, annoyed with ourselves for being so late. The woman behind the counter was calm. She kept telling Kate not to worry. The airline hadn't let us down. The departure of the flight to London was delayed by two and a half hours. Kate was asked if she needed any special assistance. She said no. When she was given her boarding card, it had 'PREG' on it. This explained the extra solicitousness.

Kate refused to be scanned by the handheld scanner. We had to wait until a senior security man decided that she wasn't a security risk, then they allowed her through without any security scans.

We had to wait two hours in the departure lounge. The metal chairs were as comfortable as scaffolding, so Kate decided she would be more comfortable lying on the floor. I bought glasses of milk from the bar to soothe her heartburn.

Every time I fly now, I think of Steve. He has refused to fly ever since he was on a plane that encountered extreme turbulence. 'You know you're in trouble when the stewardesses are screaming,' he told me. I think of that every time I take off.

As a kid, I loved aeroplanes. As a teenager, instead of women, I had aeroplanes on my wall, posters of Fokker Triplanes instead of Sam Fox. I used to be a fearless flyer. Now I'm nervous. I remind myself that the odds are in my favour. It's a million to one chance that our plane will be the one that crashes this month. In the absence of God, I trust in mathematics. I'm relying on the same statistical guardian to protect my child's well-being. Most children are born healthy. It's irrational to fear that ours won't be.

Alice kicked strongly as the plane took off. She seemed to be headbutting Kate's tummy. At last London appeared like a jewel in the night. Eight thousand feet above Hyde Park, we could see the Thames, Canary Wharf, the London Eye.

By the time we landed at Stansted, the airport was deserted, the promised ground crew were missing. The trains had stopped. We took a coach to Victoria, arriving in London at 2.40 am.

I asked Kate what it's like travelling when pregnant. She said it's important to carry wet wipes so that you can clean toilet seats. Usually she hovers over the seats in public toilets, but that's impossible when you're constipated and pregnant.

Wednesday 12 March
London is cold and grey. But on the way to Sainsbury's, I noticed signs of spring: daffodils in the park; blossom on a tree; graffiti on a street sign; a burgled car with smashed windows and no wheels. Lighter, warmer days bring out the flowers and the hooligans.

Kate said to me tonight, 'I did a nice big pooh today.'

What did we use to talk about? I replied, 'Can we talk about something else?'

She said, 'I think my belly button is going to pop out.'

An old friend phoned. I listened to Kate describing her pregnancy. She said, 'I'm really enjoying it.' She mentioned the scare about the scan, but in a casual way that minimised the distress it caused.

We tend to hide the true extent of our feelings, even from friends, even from ourselves. There are good reasons for this. The emotional vicissitudes of a single day would exhaust us if we paid attention to all of them.

I looked at the calendar. Oh my God. It's week 30.

Thursday 13 March
In the middle of the night, heartburn woke Kate up. It was like acid burning her chest and throat. I was woken by her tossing and turning, huffing and puffing. I said into the darkness, 'Is there anything I can do?'

'No.'

I was pleased by this answer because I just wanted to sleep. Moving as few parts of my body as possible, I stretched out an arm and found her spine and rubbed it soothingly in a five-second gesture of sympathy, then went back to sleep.

When Kate came home from work, she felt awful. She has read that heartburn is exacerbated by oily foods. Tonight she took no chances. Her supper consisted of a bowl of porridge and a banana.

We're both feeling burdened by the list of things we need to do before the birth. I have to write a play. I need to sand the bathroom floor. I wouldn't mind if our baby arrived late. Several months late would be handy.

A friend phoned. I wasn't in the mood for chit-chat. She could hear the preoccupation and impatience in my voice. She is a mother of two teenagers. 'Time doesn't stop just because you have a baby,' she promised me, 'you can still do things.' This is a good point. I mustn't get frantic and start regarding the baby's arrival as the end of my life. I have to stop regarding the event as if it's a terminal illness, the end of things rather than a beginning.

In order to make room for a cot, I have to dismantle a bookcase and store the beloved books in a box in the attic. It seems cruelly symbolic. But I don't mind as much as I did a few weeks ago. I'm eager to meet my daughter.

Friday 14 March
Sunny, windy, cold.

'Nice day,' I said to a neighbour when we passed in the street.

'It would be lovely,' he said, 'if I didn't have to work.'

I had another bone-cracking, muscle-crunching appointment with the osteopath, Beverley. She chatted to me while she wrenched my neck and pulverised my back. She told me how much she likes her job. If you do a job you don't enjoy, she said, it crushes your spirit. It's important to be passionate about your work, she said, because it takes up so much of your life.

She only works on Fridays. She says that she might work three days a week when her children are older, but no more than that. When I mentioned that Kate is considering working three days a week, Beverley suggested that she might not want to go back to work at all. 'Your children aren't small for long,' she explained.

I don't think Kate would want to give up work completely. She has said that. But she might want to work for fewer days. And she'll only have that option if I can earn some money.

Walking down the street, thinking about this situation, the pressure is palpable, a physical sensation, a tightness in the chest, a stiffening of limbs, a general heaviness.

Kate has been having similar thoughts to me. She came home from work and said that she was tense. 'There's so much work to do. So many cases. And so little time left.'

She is constipated again. 'I feel like I've got a piece of concrete up my bottom.'

I complimented her new red blouse. 'Nice top.'

'It makes me look huge, though.'

'It doesn't. You are huge. You can't blame the top.'

When we lie on the sofa together, watching the news, I can hardly breathe. It is my job to stroke her hair.

I wash the dishes while she gets ready for bed. She comes into the kitchen.

'Lovey, I think I've had another growth spurt.' She lifts her top and exposes her belly. It is huge. Graduating from a protuberance to an encumbrance.

Sometimes her gums bleed when she cleans her teeth.

Saturday 15 March

Kate didn't sleep well. The bones of her legs are aching. She can't find a position in bed that's comfortable for more than a minute. She was woken at 6.30 am by the baby's kicking, and couldn't get back to sleep for three hours.

The circumference of her waist has reached 100 centimetres (39½ inches).

The *linea nigra*, which has been visible for several weeks, is quite distinct now. It's a dark vertical line above and below her belly button.

Cycling towards Brockwell Park, I was nearly killed by a bus that sped through a red light. There are some complete idiots on the road. And I'm one of them. Every so often I find myself pedalling madly through a half-second gap in the traffic as lorries and taxis thunder around me. Taking these risks is even more stupid now that I'm responsible for the little one.

For lunch Kate met an old friend, Susan, whom she hasn't seen for a year. I went to join them later on Peckham Rye and found them sitting on a bench in the sun. They weren't looking at the trees or the flowers or the dogs or the passers-by. They were staring at Kate's exposed belly, waiting for the baby to kick. I was concerned that Kate's friend might not find this as entertaining as we do, but she claimed to be fascinated. None of Susan's friends has children, so she has never had the opportunity of closely examining the freakish curiosity that is a pregnant woman. The baby, who was kicking like a donkey this morning, disappointed her audience by sleeping all afternoon.

Friends can't resist trying to guess the baby's name. They all have particular theories. Susan thinks we'll choose something 'exotic' and 'fancy' and 'musical-sounding' such as Anastasia. Not something 'Middle England' like Hannah or Emily.

Kate's ankles are swollen. There's an indentation when she takes her socks off.

Sunday 16 March   Week 31

Claude and Denise came round for lunch. The good thing about having visitors is that it makes you clean your house.

Kate had baked a quiche. My contributions were olive bread and a black-currant cake – the product of my own hands, which had carried them from Peckham Farmers' Market this morning.

They arrived with Thierry, who is four months old now. When he smiles, he looks like a carp.

His parents generously shared their mistakes and tips with us. In the early weeks of Thierry's life, they gave him medicine thinking he was complaining of colic, until they realised that he was just hungry.

As a parent you have to learn to do everything with one hand. Claude was slicing bread while holding his son under his other arm. He stopped slicing when he noticed blood. Somehow the baby's hand had got in the way. Luckily he only suffered a minor cut near the wrist, rather than complete amputation.

We couldn't begin our lunch until Thierry had finished his. This took a while. I waited patiently. Then I waited impatiently. Nobody else seemed to mind. A feeding baby is a spectator sport. Our food went cold while we waited for Thierry to drink his milk and swallow his mushy carrot.

Normally Claude talks incessantly. Today it is Denise who never shuts up. I've never seen her like this before. It's as if she has been in prison for four months. She keeps saying how relaxing it is to be given lunch instead of providing it.

Denise looks at her baby with the adoration of a disciple. It is slightly off-putting. Is that what's going to happen to us? Are we going to be drugged and brainwashed, the victims of hormones and childcare gurus? I felt a brief resurgence of my old fears. Parenthood is a sect.

If we fall short of perfection in our parenting skills, it's good to know that we won't be alone. I've discovered the Bad Mothers Club (www. badmothersclub.co.uk), a website that allows parents to tell the truth about their lives. There's a section entitled 'Tantrum of the Week': 'I was giving the kids their dinner and they wouldn't eat any of it. They just whined for biscuits the whole time. Finally, I got so sick of it, I took the last packet out of the cupboard, jumped up and down on it, and threw it in the bin.' These true tales are an antidote to the idealism of the childcare experts in the pregnancy magazines. There's an article about bedtimes. 'One pet theory is that children "find their own bedtimes". Sure! Like they find their own vegetables!'

Monday 17 March

Last week, for the umpteenth time, I left a message on the midwife's answerphone asking her to confirm the dates of the NHS parentcraft classes. We have heard nothing from her, so we decided to go along tonight to the scheduled appointment.

Kate rushed home from work and wolfed down her pasta so we wouldn't be late. She brought along a small rucksack with almost nothing in it, just a notebook and a couple of pens. I insisted on carrying it. It looks bad if your pregnant partner is carrying all the luggage.

Under a bright moon, we walked to Dulwich Hospital for our first Parent Education class. The door was locked, the lights were off, there was nobody there. We checked our letter. It was the correct time, the correct day, the correct hospital. There was nobody around who could explain the mystery. So we just went home again. Kate was peeved. 'It just makes me angry.' Our faith in NHS competence wasn't helped when we walked past a noticeboard in the hospital. I hope their nursing is better than their spelling. Syringes had been spelt 'srynges'.

Tuesday 18 March

Another day, another hospital. We had an antenatal appointment at 9.30 am. Kate told me last week that I don't have to come if I don't want to. But I want to. It makes me feel that I'm contributing to my child's out-bringing. I like hearing the heartbeat.

We get a different midwife every time. This time it was a woman whose badge said 'Annette'. She was the most efficient and organised of all the midwives we've met. She had a baby five months ago, so perhaps she is more conscious of how pregnant women like to be treated. She was patient, clear and unpatronising.

Kate's blood pressure has changed, but remains within the acceptable range.

'Is the baby moving a lot?' asked Annette.

'Yes,' said Kate, 'but some days more than others.'

'You can prod it. Not a gentle tap, a firm prod. Or you can turn over onto your other side and see if that makes the baby move. If you're worried, phone the hospital. Day or night. They'll tell you to come in and they'll monitor the baby's heart.'

Annette says that Kate should be able to detect the baby's movements about 10 times in a 10–12 hour period. Nobody has told us this before. Maybe it's better not to know. Now we're going to start counting and worrying.

Annette tried to listen to the baby's heartbeat with a handheld monitor the size of a mobile phone. Kate's belly sounded like the depths of the ocean. But we couldn't find the heartbeat. Then we heard it: faint, weak, distant, as if the baby was hiding on the seabed. It was beating 143 times every minute.

Annette says that the baby should start to turn soon. Kate ought to feel 'more pressure down below' as the baby turns its head towards the exit.

Annette looked on the computer at 'the bloods', the results of the routine blood tests that Kate had a month ago.

'Have you been feeling tired?'

'No,' said Kate. 'I've had quite a lot of energy.'

'It's just that your iron level is slightly below the normal range.' She went to find some iron supplements but there were none in stock. Instead she told us to eat more greens. 'I'm not alarmed,' said Annette. This made us alarmed.

Outside the hospital, we waited for a bus. Kate said that she felt tired. 'But we eat lots of greens,' she said.

'We're meant to eat five portions of fruit and vegetables every day.'

'I do.'

'How many did you have yesterday?'

'Two.'

'What did you have for lunch yesterday?'

'A roll with Philadelphia cheese. And a doughnut.'

I went to the supermarket and bought half a tonne of green vegetables and fruit.

Wednesday 19 March

This morning we walked to the hospital for yet another scan. Kate has been so optimistic about everything. She says that she has the advantage of having the baby inside her, so she can feel that everything is all right, whereas I can't.

Her positive outlook has affected me and I have been regarding the prospect of the scan with a superficial confidence. But in my heart of hearts I am afraid for the baby.

We were processed by people we'd never seen before. The sonographer was an Eastern European woman who pronounced Kate's name 'Cat-a'. In a dimly lit room, Kate lay down and I sat in a chair next to the bed. The sonographer operated the ultrasound machine and read out the measurements to another woman who tapped the figures into a computer.

Kate looked at me worriedly when we heard the figure 'eleven point eight'. This meant that the ventricle had enlarged in size.

Later a female consultant joined us and checked the measurements. The first woman had made a mistake. She had measured incorrectly. The ventricle measurement was 'nine point nine'.

It hasn't got worse after all. The ventricle still looks prominent but other parts of the brain look normal. The consultant mumbled all this to her colleagues. She wasn't talking to us at all. They were behaving as if we weren't there. The consultant mentioned to her assistants that she intends to send Kate for an MRI scan.

'What's the purpose of that?' asked Kate.

'I'll explain it all later,' said the consultant brusquely.

Meanwhile other people were entering the room and gathering to look at the ultrasound machine. This is a teaching hospital. We are an interesting case. Kate was facing the wall so she couldn't see the crowd gathering behind her. She was taken aback when she finally noticed the eight people standing behind her head. The consultant printed out some images of our baby's brain. A mob gathered around it eagerly.

Eventually the consultant spoke to us. She explained that an MRI scan reveals elements of the brain invisible to ultrasound. It might reveal some bleeding in the brain, which may explain the prominence of the ventricles. The magnetic resonance imaging has no harmful side effects, she told us.

So in the end we agreed to have the MRI scan in a couple of weeks. If it finds that everything is normal, we won't have to worry quite so much.

As we left the room, the mob was still surrounding the picture of our baby's brain, pointing and whispering. Kate had to fight her way past them to get to her coat. 'Bye,' I said, aiming for the lightest touch of sarcasm. 'Bye,' they chorused, remembering their manners. Nobody had asked us if we objected to eight strangers intruding on our private discussions.

I have that feeling of dread again. Kate went to work. I walked home and ate chocolate. My mood is veering between an awful fear of being lumbered with a disabled child – and I feel ashamed of that feeling – and a sentimental determination to love it unconditionally.

The truth is, I don't know what's going to happen or how I'm going to feel. A relationship is a leap of faith. In times of difficulty, you not only trust your partner to do the right thing, you put faith in yourself to do the right thing.

When you decide to have kids, you know it's going to be hard work. But you also have an expectation that the rewards make it worthwhile. A severely disabled child might be unable to participate in many of the pleasures a parent has been looking forward to. What's the answer? The answer is to love your child exactly as she is. I hope I can do that. I worry what kind of person my child is going to be. I also worry about what kind of person I'm going to be.

On Wednesday evenings, Kate has piano lessons. She is practising for her grade-four exam. Tonight her piano teacher suggested that she should abandon the piece of music she has been trying to learn. The teacher thinks that Kate hasn't got the 'mental agility' to cope with this piece of music while she's pregnant.

Kate doesn't think that she is lacking in mental agility. She asked me what I think. I said, as nicely as possible, that there have been moments when she hasn't been as sharp as she'd normally be.

Tonight I phoned Sarah for a chat. She is expecting her fourth child. By coincidence, she asked if Kate's brain is still working properly. Sarah confessed that she herself exists in a state of extreme stupidity when she's pregnant. 'I shock myself with my stupidity,' she admitted. She started to tell me about a book she was reading last night, but she couldn't remember the title. She said, 'You see what I mean?'

Sarah predicts that we'll be deliriously happy when our first baby is born. 'You'll feel special. The first two weeks were the most golden and special I can remember. And it's never ever the same again.'

Thursday 20 March

Everyone's story is different. I asked another friend, a mother of two teenage children, if the first two weeks after the birth of her first child were the most golden and special of her life. They weren't. She 'didn't bond immediately' with her son. After five days, she burst into tears. 'After five days,' she said, 'everyone bursts into tears. It's a scientific fact.' And then there was a period 'when the hormones kicked in' and she wanted to have ten babies. She 'wanted to populate the world' because babies seemed so wonderful. There was more unconditional joy surrounding the birth of her second child because, having experienced the delightfulness of babies, 'we loved her before she was born'. And then she said what everyone says: 'It's the best thing I've ever done.'

'You're not dead yet.'

'I don't think I'll ever top that.'

People's stories aren't just different from other people's. They are different from themselves. Moments after acclaiming the joy of babies, my friend said that she prefers older children. 'The baby bit is wonderful for about two hours a day. But the rest of it is drudgery.'

We love our baby already. We talk to her every day. At least, I love my idea of her. After she is born, if she is very different from my preconceptions of her, I wonder if I will love her as much? Will the hormones kick in? Is that all love is – a hormone surge? The Greek and Hebrew languages have several different words for love in all its variety. Sanskrit has 96. Persian has 80. We are about to learn a new kind of love.

Cycled from Peckham to Leicester Square. It was rush hour. Car drivers were in a mad frenzy trying to get home. London is plagued by mad car disease. The journey involved about ten near-death experiences and an altercation with a teenager. For a laugh, he pretended to ram my bike with his bike, only swerving away at the last second. I suggested that he should show people more respect, but slightly undermined my own argument by calling him an arsehole.

Met a friend and we went to see a film on Tottenham Court Road. All our friends are amazed that we've been put through intense anxiety and intimate examination just because one measurement was slightly above the normal range. It's true that no other hospital in the country would be subjecting us to this. Only King's Hospital has the equipment to detect or the data to assess this particular statistical anomaly. I don't know if we are beneficiaries or victims of modern medicine. It has changed our experience of the pregnancy. I am enjoying it less. And I fear that it will alter my relationship with my child. As I watch my daughter grow up, I don't want to be studying her for signs of learning disability.

Kate has borrowed a stethoscope from work. She has to take it back in the morning. By the time I got home, it was too late. She was asleep.

Friday 21 March

Kate woke me up and attached the stethoscope to my ears. Dimly I could hear our baby's heart beating. Then I listened to Kate's heart beating. Then I listened to my own heart beating. Satisfied that we are all alive and well, I went back to sleep.

More warnings of things to come. I was chatting to Louise on the phone. She told me about the tacit rivalry among parents. Her friends' children went to private schools but haven't done as well as her own two children who went to state schools and who are studying at Oxford and Cambridge now. Louise can't help feeling gratified by this comparison.

I hate this parental competitiveness that turns children into status symbols. It's a disease I hope not to catch.

But I'm already showing the first symptoms. I will be disappointed if our child is thick. Sorry – has learning difficulties. I am uncomfortable with these feelings. I feel hypocritical. It must've been a shock for my mum when I emerged from the womb with a cleft lip and palate. I probably wasn't the kind of baby she'd imagined. But I was loved unreservedly.

Obviously I'd like a bright and responsive child but, after the scan results, I'm scared to hope for that now.

Your child is someone, like your partner, with whom you'll share your home and the rest of your life. Your partner is the result of a selection process lasting years, whereas your child is just a lucky dip.

And you're stuck with them for life. The more I think about it, the more I think the best thing is not to think about it. But the mind can't be turned off. The mind has thoughts like the heart has beats.

Our baby is lying with her head downwards, ready for birth. A thought has occurred to Kate. 'If we have sex, does your penis touch the baby's head?' We looked at diagrams in a book. It doesn't. But it looks close enough to jolt the baby. Now we're even less likely to have sex.

As Kate gets bigger, I am becoming more useful. It's my job to get things from the top shelf. Lentils. Rice.

She regularly mentions her weight, even though her friends keep telling her that she hasn't put any on. She looks more or less the same, apart from the bump itself.

Lay on the sofa, watching sitcoms, feeling the baby kicking wildly. Kate says cuddling on the sofa is one of her favourite things. When women say 'cuddling', they mean 'being cuddled'.

I was reading Kaz Cooke's diary in *The Rough Guide to Pregnancy & Birth*. In week 31 she writes, 'Not much more to buy now.' We haven't bought anything yet.

Saturday 22 March

I was in the middle of peeing when Kate appeared at the loo door with a crumpled tearful face. I was frightened but tried not to show it. What was wrong? Was she bleeding? I stopped what I was doing and told her that it was OK, even though I didn't know what it was.

'Eight thousand babies die at birth or soon after birth,' she said. 'I don't think I should read those books any more.' She had been browsing through *The Pregnancy Book* issued by the NHS to expectant mothers.

She is starting to worry about things that can go wrong. She says that she's glad she's so busy at work. It gives her less time to be anxious.

The books are still useful for some things. Kate has read that, by this stage of pregnancy, it's possible to hear the baby's heartbeat with the naked ear. So I put my ear to her belly and there it was. A loud, fast, beating heart. When I spoke to the baby, the heartbeat seemed to beat faster and louder. Maybe I was imagining that. I was delighted to have some connection with the baby.

Kate phoned my mum today to ask about hyacinths. My mum said on the phone, 'Oh I'd love to be there and see that little baby coming out.' Kate told me afterwards, 'I didn't say anything. I just ignored it. I felt a bit bad. I don't know if it was a hint.'

I'm sure it was a hint. I said, 'Do you want her there?'

'No. Do you want her there?'

'No. I'd feel a bit inhibited. I'd rather it was just the two of us.'

The two of us and a horde of obstetric staff. One of my friends gave permission for students to observe her giving birth. They have to learn, she told herself. In the midst of a painful labour, she changed her mind. She turned to the students and said, 'You lot, fuck off!' And they fucked off.

My mum advised Kate to remove her rings at the first sign of swelling. When my mum was pregnant, the rings had to be cut off her engorged fingers. (She still has the severed rings, a memento of the pregnancy, and also a symbol of her severance from her carefree youth.)

Kate slid her ring on and off her finger as a test. Being so active, walking so much, has helped to minimise some of the discomforts. She thinks she would've suffered much more from fluid retention and backache. She looks like her usual self, but with a bump. Some of the pregnant women in the waiting rooms at the hospital look like puffer fish.

Later I found Kate crying on the sofa. It was time for another hug. She said, 'I don't really know why I'm crying.'

She was tired and tearful all evening. Her ribs above the bump felt sore. We were both in a grumpy mood. She said, 'At least I've got a good reason.'

'What reason?'

'I'm pregnant. It's biology.'

'What am I, clockwork?'

Sunday 23 March   Week 32

In bed I placed my ear against the bump and tried to listen to the baby. She has moved. I found her heartbeat, fast and regular, on the other side.

A sociable afternoon. We went to Walthamstow to have lunch with Louise. She said to Kate, 'Are you happy with it? Because I felt like I had an alien inside me.' Kate doesn't feel like the baby is a parasite.

When Louise's contractions started, she was visiting her mother. Her mother wasn't insured to drive the car, so Louise had to drive herself 50 miles to the hospital, from Gloucester to Bristol. During the labour, her husband suggested that she should squeeze his hand when it was painful. Somehow, squeezing his hand didn't seem sufficient for the degree of pain, so she punched him in the stomach.

A sociable evening. We went to Tufnell Park to have supper with friends. Everyone asked Kate how she is feeling. These people told jollier, more con- soling stories about childbirth. One of them has heard that it's merely like 'bad period pains'. None of them has children.

Two of our friends have relatives in India. They told us that Indian women go to bed for 40 days after the birth of their child and, throughout this period, they are pampered by the rest of the family. Kate would like to introduce this tradition to South London.

Monday 24 March

Kate is planning to work until two weeks before the birth. This allows her more maternity leave after the baby is born. Tonight she got home from work earlier than usual, about six o'clock, and lay on the sofa.

'How are you feeling?' I said.

'Need a rest.'

She looked worried. 'She's not moving. She hasn't moved much all day.' I listened to her belly and heard Alice's heartbeat. 'She's fine.' During the evening, Kate felt her moving.

We've decided that we're glad that we know the sex of our baby after all. It allows us to address her by name. It brings her closer.

We trekked to Emma and Simon's house in Tooting for supper. Emma chopped a few carrots, then Simon took over in the kitchen while Emma chatted to Kate. I felt humbled by Simon's culinary prowess. This is what I should be like, I thought, cooking while Kate chats to her friends. Then the food arrived and I didn't feel so bad. The couscous was dry; it was like eating sand. The chocolate sauce ('I must've taken my eye off it,' said Simon) was lumpy, like dog shit.

When their daughter was born, their cat ran away. It came back after a week, but can still be a bit sulky.

It wasn't only the cat's feelings that were complicated. Emma said candidly that it was two months before she could describe her feelings for her baby as love.

We picked up some more useful tips. 'If you go to a restaurant with your baby, choose pasta rather than pizza. It's easier to eat with one hand.'

Kate accused me of looking depressed. It was because many of their anecdotes about parenthood are tales of misery and mayhem. They said they can only do anything for ten minutes at a time before they're called away. Both parents are permanently tired. Simon said, 'One of the strange things about having kids is that suddenly you crave the company of your in-laws. You appreciate anyone who's willing to liberate you from childminding duties for a while so you can sleep and have a peaceful moment for yourself.'

They noticed the look on my face. Emma said, 'It's tough but it's wonderful. It's all worth it.'

Tuesday 25 March

I haven't felt the craving yet, but I can see that the baby's grandparents are already circling. Kate phoned from work to confirm that her mother is coming to visit next weekend. She also said, 'Everyone is amazed that I'm having the baby at the end of May.'

'Why?'

'Because they think I'm so small.'

'They haven't seen you naked.'

'That's true.'

One of my jobs is to reassure her that she is healthily big. Then she starts asking: 'Am I fat?'

The people across the road look after their grandson when their daughter goes to work. I've never spoken to any of them, beyond an occasional 'hello', but they are a tiny part of my life. I've seen this little boy regularly since he was a small baby. Today I saw him walking down the steps, holding his granny's hand. It was like a miracle. It was wonderful and perturbing at the same time. It left me amazed at the efficiency of life's processes, unnerved by the speed and relentlessness of change.

I've found a small lump in my mouth, quite sore. Naturally my first thought was: mouth cancer, I'm going to die.

I played football in Brixton. In the pub afterwards, we talked about babies. Half of the players are dads now. Bobby gave me a sanguine view of fatherhood. He said, 'The first three months are a shit storm, but then things calm down. Or you calm down.' He also said, 'If the woman is amenable, it's still possible for the man to have an unimpeded life.'

I don't think I've ever had an unimpeded life. There's always something getting in the way of something.

Wednesday 26 March

In the middle of the night, Kate got angry at the bed sheet entangled around her leg. When we woke up she apologised for being grumpy, and then continued to be grumpy.

On the doormat, a gas bill *and* an electricity bill.

I phoned my producers to find out how much progress they've made. Very little. They are bickering among themselves about the size of their own fees.

This afternoon I met a friend who revealed that she has just had a miscarriage. She was seven weeks pregnant. That's the second time in two days someone has told me that they've had a miscarriage recently. It reminds me that this process is a life and death struggle. Our baby has done well to get this far.

Kate has felt 'a different kind of feeling', a sharp twinge in her lower abdomen. She thinks it might be Braxton Hicks contractions. Braxton Hicks is another addition to our vocabulary. They are slight contractions of the uterus that occur throughout pregnancy. Most women don't notice them until the third trimester when they are often mistaken for labour. *NCT Complete Book of Pregnancy* says on page 168 that these tightenings of the muscles of the womb are 'not painful', but the same book says on page 70 that they 'may be quite painful'.

Alice is kicking more strongly these days. She booted me in the cheek tonight when I was listening to her heart beating.

Thursday 27 March
We met at the hospital. Kate was fairly cheerful.

An MRI scan uses magnetism to display parts of the body undetected by ultrasound. 'You're not allowed into the scanning room with any metal objects,' explained the operator, a rotund Irishman with smiling eyes and a soothing, charming, southern Irish accent. I told him that I have screws and wires in my jaw from old operations, but he said that I should be safe. It's loose objects that can fly across the room.

Kate was given headphones to protect her ears from the noise of the scanner. Through the headphones she could hear a radio station, occasionally interrupted by the operator's voice. She was given a lemon-shaped rubber capsule to hold in her left hand. It was an emergency button.

'Squeeze that if you want us,' said the nice Irishman.

'Why would I want you?' asked Kate innocently.

I already knew the answer to this. My mum had a MRI scan many years ago. For some people it can be a terrifying, claustrophobic experience. That's not how the Irishman explained it. But he did say, 'At least once a day we have somebody who decides it's not for them, and they stand up and walk out.'

'How long will it be?' she asked.

'Well, that kind of depends on the little one. If she's quiet and still, it might be twenty minutes, but if she's moving around, it might take forty minutes.'

Kate was strapped onto a tray, which lifted and slid into a narrow white cylinder. A plastic mesh was placed over her belly. She disappeared into the machine, feet first, until I could only see the top of her head.

'Are you all right, lovey?'

'Yeah.'

It was a snug fit; she was like a tampon inside a tampon applicator. The wall of the cylinder was an inch above her nose. I sat on a chair outside the machine, looking at her hair. There was a pair of headphones for me as well. The Irishman said that I may or may not need them. He left the room. The scan began. For a few seconds the machine made a deafening noise, like an alarm on a military airbase.

Then there was a silence. Then there was a different kind of shrillness, like a siren. Then there was a silence. This sequence of sirens and silence continued for several minutes. In a moment of quietness, I said, 'Are you all right, lovey?'

'No,' she said.

This wasn't the answer I was expecting. At that moment the Irishman walked into the scanning room. I wasn't expecting that either. He pressed a button. The tray began to move and Kate slid out of the machine like an ejected videotape.

'Are you OK?' he asked her. Kate had pressed the emergency button.

'My belly's hot,' she said, distress in her voice.

'I've not heard that before,' said the Irishman.

'It's hot on my belly. It feels like it's in direct sunlight.'

The Irishman's eyes weren't smiling. They glanced at me. I said, 'Are you OK, lovey? It's meant to be completely safe for the baby.' Meanwhile the Irishman briefly checked the equipment, the tubes and the plastic mesh, and pronounced that everything was normal. Not entirely reassured, Kate consented to continue with the scan. She slid back into the machine.

I said, 'Don't worry, lovey. I was reading about it this morning. It's meant to be completely safe.' Actually, the medical reports phrase it carefully. There's no evidence that it causes any harm, they say. There's a small theoretical risk to a developing foetus so women aren't scanned during the first 12 weeks of pregnancy.

The scan recommenced. The loud noises returned. The machine doesn't sound harmless.

After a couple of minutes, the Irishman came into the room. Kate had pressed the emergency button again. As she was ejected from the machine, she said: 'I need to go to the toilet.' The Irishman extricated her from the apparatus. I helped her to sit up. She was hot. Her skin was clammy, her hair was straggly with sweat.

I guided her towards the toilet. 'Do you want me to come in with you?'

'Yeah.'

Inside the toilet, she tried to cool down and calm down. She told me what she had heard through the headphones. The first time she pressed the emergency button, she heard a woman's voice say calmly, 'We're coming.' The second time she pressed the button, the same woman's voice had said plaintively, 'Just one more image.'

I kissed her forehead and stroked her hair and told her not to worry. I repeated the advice I'd read. It's meant to be completely safe. I don't know if there was total conviction in my voice.

When we emerged from the toilet, the nice Irishman told us that the scan was completed and she didn't need to go into the machine again. 'Are you sure?' she asked. She'd only been in there for ten minutes. 'Five seconds sooner and it wouldn't have been,' he said cheerfully. I asked, 'Have you got all the images you need?' He assured us that he did. We weren't completely convinced, but we didn't argue.

Kate was apologetic about causing a fuss. She hadn't been bothered by the prospect of the scan. She hadn't expected to feel like that. It felt as if she was being microwaved.

Outside the sun was shining. We walked through Ruskin Park. Kate said, 'That's the nearest I've ever come to a panic attack. I thought my head was going to explode. It was horrible. It was horrible.'

We have to wait nearly two weeks for the results.

Friday 28 March
It isn't mouth cancer. It's an abscess. The doctor has prescribed antibiotics. The right side of my face is sore and swollen. I look like a chipmunk. It serves me right for saying that pregnant women look like puffer fish.

Kate now regrets telling my mum that she was going to have the MRI scan. It has provoked unnecessary anxiety and unwanted interest. My mum phoned today to ask how it went. Kate admitted that it was 'a worse experience than I anticipated. Really noisy and really hot. It was a feeling like intense sunshine. And I thought, what if there's something wrong with the machine and it's harming the baby? I felt really hot and, I suppose, claustrophobic. Like I couldn't breathe. And I thought, what's it like for the baby if the mother's feeling so tense?'

My mum told Kate not to worry about the baby's prognosis. Kate found this irritating as well. She feels that the baby is going to be fine. She resents being consoled about things she's not worried about.

'Oooh!' said Kate. 'Aaaaah!' said Kate. A couple of times she was surprised by the force of the baby's kicks. Her body has become like one of those toys that makes different noises when a child presses the various parts of it. When the baby pushes, Kate makes a noise. The baby was pushing so hard that Kate thought her belly button was going to pop out.

Kate can't see anything below her belly button.

Feeling scared during yesterday's scan, she says, has made her think about how she'll cope at the birth. She wonders if she is underestimating the 'trauma and difficulty' of it.

I've had the same thought. For many women, childbirth is the first time they've encountered extreme physical anguish. I'm guessing that it's worse than a leg wax. I fear that we'll concoct a birth plan that excludes major painkillers and epidurals, and then the agonising reality of the labour will change Kate's mind, and we'll end up haggling in the maternity ward. I'll be saying, 'But you said you only wanted gas and air. Look, it's here, in writing.' And she'll be saying, 'Give me the fucking drugs, you bastard!' I fear that it's not going to be a serene or dignified occasion.

Over the weeks, Kate's nipples have been slowly darkening. Now the areolae are almost black. Fried eggs of dark chocolate. The change in colour gives the baby a clear target when it's hungry.

Saturday 29 March

It hasn't always been like this. Kate phoned her Yorkshire granny, Harriet.

Harriet says that she's always surprised when she sees images of women screaming during childbirth. 'We never made that much noise.'

When Harriet was pregnant in the 1940s with her second child – Kate's uncle – she was living in Hong Kong. There were regular typhoons and, as each storm approached, Harriet was moved to the other side of the island to be nearer the hospital. She got bored with this constant upheaval so she decided to get herself admitted to hospital early. She faked her labour pains. In the hospital, when the baby failed to arrive, the doctors induced the birth using a combination of 'castor oil and brandy'.

A while ago I took a photo of Kate and her pregnant sister-in-law standing back to back on Brighton beach. Kate sent a copy of this photo to her granny who remarked that Kate's great-granny would've been 'shocked' to see the two expectant mothers 'flaunting your bumps'.

The baby is trying to punch her way out. The dome of Kate's belly turned into a pyramid, a giant piece of white Toblerone.

Sunday 30 March Week 33

We woke up early. The baby was restless and so was her mother. Kate suggested we should tell people that we'll get the MRI scan results on Thursday 10 April. I agreed. In fact, we'll get them two days before. She says this will give us extra time to get used to the implications if the scan finds something amiss in the baby's brain. Otherwise some people will phone the same day. We might not be in the mood to talk to them. We might be upset. Kate said all this in her normal calm voice. Then tears erupted and her face crumpled.

I don't know what benefit we're getting from this medical attention. If there hadn't been such a detailed second scan, if our baby hadn't been factored and subtracted by the medical algebra, we would be enjoying a 'normal' pregnancy.

Today is Mother's Day. I gave Kate a card and a present. Inside the card it says:

> My love,
> Congratulations on your first Mother's Day.
> We love you lots.
> XXX XXX

The last three kisses were written in the baby's wobbly handwriting. This is the kind of thing that has always annoyed me.

I used to get irritated when I saw babies wearing T-shirts with slogans like 'I Love My Mum'. It seemed like the peak of parental presumption and vanity. Now I'm participating in the same charade. I'm putting words in the baby's mouth, and have been for months, anthropomorphising a cluster of cells, projecting thoughts and feelings onto an amorphous fruit-sized embryo. It's the beginning of the process of indoctrinating the child into social and familial habits. And a way of indoctrinating and indulging ourselves. Until the child can speak for herself, she is like a doll with whom we have imaginary conversations.

We had visitors for the afternoon. My mum and stepfather and their dog, Alfie. The dog was so excited that he peed on my shoe. Kate was revolted. Later she told me, 'I don't like dogs that pee on you and slobber on you. He's so exhausting.' 'Wait till you have a baby,' I told her.

My mum admired the bump. Then she looked at Kate's bottom and said, 'You're not that bad at the back.' She meant to be kind. Noticing that Kate was disconcerted by this uninvited assessment of her rear end, my mum added reassuringly, 'No, I've seen some pregnant women who are huge there.' Kate looked at me and I widened my eyes, trying to find an expression that would simultaneously convey outrage, helplessness and stoicism.

I gave Kate a present. It's a book she wanted. *What To Expect: The First Year.* It has 662 pages. Flipping through the index reveals Vomiting, Words, Weaning, Teething, Seizures, Spitup, Pinkeye, Mothering (boredom with), Illnesses, Grilled Cheese Sandwich, Flat Feet, Drooling, Dog Bites, Crying, Colic, Burping, Accidents to Baby.

The topic on page 280 of *What To Expect*, according to the index, is Masturbation. This prospect depresses me. I turned to page 280 and discovered that the authors were talking about children playing with their genitals, not parents. But they do warn elsewhere that 'most women find the post-partum period (and sometimes a several-month stretch following it) a sexual wasteland'.

Monday 31 March

The nature of the birth can have long-term consequences for the child and the mother. Post-natal depression is more common among mothers who feel a loss of control during the birth as a result of interventions by medical staff. Many forms of pain relief have side effects on the mother and/or the baby. Some drugs adversely affect the baby's ability to breastfeed, which can have significant implications for its development. Excessive medicalisation of the birth experience can turn the positive aspects of an amazing life event into a distressing ordeal. Birth is always a drama, but it needn't be a trauma. So there are good reasons for pregnant parents to be interested in the kind of birth being offered to them.

Once again we walked to Dulwich Hospital for our first Parent Education class. We wrote our names on sticky labels and stuck them to our chests. We sat in a semicircle. There were 15 of us. Eight women and seven men. The midwife leading the group was Yvonne. She made us introduce ourselves. The women had to state their name and their due date. The men had to say how they felt about becoming a father. The first man said he was 'excited and nervous'. After that, all the men said they were 'excited and nervous'.

Then we were divided into three smaller groups and told to make a list of the things we wanted to know. Each group wrote the same thing at the top of the list. 'Pain relief'.

Some of my friends with kids had warned me that these classes are boring and useless. In fact, it was fascinating. Yvonne stood at the front holding a plastic pelvis and a doll and explained how babies are born.

She invited us all to ask questions at any time. A man raised his hand. The first query on the subject of childbirth was: 'Where do you park?'

Yvonne told us that it's advisable to have our babies on Sundays or at night when parking is free.

One man asked if, after driving his wife to the maternity building, he would have time to take the car home and walk back to the hospital. He estimated that this would take an hour and a half. Another man suggested that we could all park in Sainsbury's free car park, which is only 20 minutes away. The first man said that this idea was 'inspired'.

Then we discussed secondary details such as the actual labour and birth. Any baby born between weeks 37 and 42 is regarded as full term. Or, as Yvonne put it, 'fully cooked'. Or, after week 40, 'slightly overcooked'. She told the women in the room to start carrying their medical notes with them at all times, just in case there was a need to go to hospital immediately.

A woman called GERALDINE asked, 'How do we know when to go to the hospital?' It's important that we don't go there straight away because we'll just be sent home again, said Yvonne. She has seen the disappointment on the faces of parents who've been turned away.

The first irregular contractions can continue for hours. Or days. Or several days. Eventually these contractions, lasting for 45 seconds or more, should become regular and painful. When the regular contractions begin, we should go for a walk, talk to friends, have a bath, do something to take our minds off it. 'Play a computer game?' suggested GARY helpfully. Yvonne said the important thing is not to dwell on it. Walk, relax and don't forget to eat. 'Birth is a marathon and you wouldn't run a marathon without eating beforehand.'

High carbohydrate foods, mixed with protein, are best. Pasta. Rice. Fish. Egg and toast. Bananas.

'Do not eat fatty food,' said Yvonne, 'do not eat fried chicken. Do not eat curry. I know a woman who ate curry before she went into labour. I've never in my life seen so much curry vomit.'

Yvonne asked if we've considered using massage as a way of relaxing between the contractions. GARY claimed that he has 'magic hands'. Everyone laughed.

If the pregnant woman finds a jelly-like substance on her knickers, this is the 'show', the mucus plug. It's like mucus from your nose but it should be clear.

When the contractions are occurring every three to five minutes, then we can consider going to the hospital. We still have a fair amount of time. They won't keep you on the labour ward until your cervix is at least 3 centimetres dilated. The baby can be born when the cervix is 10 centimetres dilated. The average rate of dilation is ½ centimetre–1 centimetre per hour. So the average length of labour for a first baby is 12–14 hours. 'Your labour won't last five days,' Yvonne assures us.

If your waters break, go to hospital immediately. If you're not sure, smell it. Your waters smell very different from urine. Normally your waters don't break until you are 8 centimetres–10 centimetres dilated, quite late in the labour. This surprises us. It's common knowledge that the breaking of the waters is a sign that a woman is going into labour. Like a lot of common knowledge, it isn't true. In most cases, the breaking of the waters occurs fairly late in the process.

TRACY asked Yvonne, 'At what point would you go into the hospital?'

Yvonne said, 'I personally would have a home birth.'

GARY explained why his partner isn't having a home birth. 'We don't want to make a mess of the carpets.'

'Can I feel when I'm dilated?' asked JENNY.

'No, and don't try,' said Yvonne.

'Will I be able to see it?' asked MIKE.

'No, not unless you've got a telescope.'

Another sign of imminent labour is rectal pressure, the feeling that you want to pooh.

Each couple had a particular anxiety. One woman asked about Strep B, a postnatal infection. Her friend's baby died shortly after birth because of Strep B.

GARY looked worried. He raised a hand. 'This poohing thing. Do all women pooh?'

'No.'

He looked relieved.

Your experience of the birth largely depends on the position of the baby. The ideal position, from the mother's point of view, is when the baby is head down with its back on the left. Most babies start to 'engage' – move into position – between weeks 34 and 36. During this period, Yvonne says, pregnant women shouldn't drive too much because car seats mean that your knees are above your hips, and this posture deters the baby from engaging. For the same reason pregnant women should sit forward rather than lean back when sitting in a chair.

The position of the baby is important because it determines which part of the baby's head emerges first. If it's in the right position, the average baby's skull has a diameter of 9½ millimetres. If it's in an awkward position, the skull's diameter can be 13½ millimetres. This is a significant difference considering that the diameter of the mother's cervix will be 10 millimetres.

Babies in the wrong position are more common now than a hundred years ago. It's because we live such sedentary lives, says Yvonne. She advises the women to 'keep mobile, walk as much as you can, drive as little as you can, wear flat shoes, sit forward, or lie on your side, don't lounge back'.

All the woman shifted in their seats and leant forward.

A final question. Is there any way we can accelerate the process, encourage the labour along? Yvonne said we can have 'lots of sex' or 'nipple stimulation'. GARY looked pleased about this. His wife pulled a face.

Tuesday 1 April
Another evening, another hospital, another midwife. This time we went to the maternity unit at King's to hear the consultant midwife talk about birthing pools.

Annie, a large woman draped in a maroon dress and a silky scarf, told us that labour in water is more relaxing for the mother and that babies born in water tend to be less distressed. They cry less, sometimes not at all.

People asked the obvious questions. Why doesn't the baby drown? Because the lungs don't operate until the baby makes contact with the air. How many pools are there? King's has two, a portable pool and a plumbed-in pool. When we go into labour, what are the chances that both pools will be occupied? That's very unlikely, said Annie.

She was evangelical about birthing pools. 'It's lovely to see. It's really wonderful.' As she said this, we were standing in the hall. The door to one of the birthing rooms was open. The sound of an animal in pain was coming from that room. Annie was still talking but nobody was listening to her. The sound of the woman giving birth was captivating, unnerving. Nobody looked anybody in the eye. Annie closed the door but we could still hear the moans, the sounds of extreme distress.

Nobody said anything, but there was some nervous giggling. As we left the ward at the end of the tour, the moaning was the only topic of conversation.

'Did that freak you out?' said a pregnant woman. 'It freaked me out. It was an animal noise.'

Kate said to me as we walked home, 'It's important to have controlled breathing, and not be frightened.' It's a good theory.

Wednesday 2 April

A letter from a friend, a mother of three. She urges me to tell Kate to reject the more invasive procedures. 'Tell her to say *no* to vaginal examinations or at least cut down to the last moment, they are the worst bit, no one did that to me after L was born!'

This is a recurring issue. Who is in charge of the pregnancy? The pregnant woman, or the medical establishment?

At the water birth seminar last night, I asked the consultant midwife about this issue of decision-making. I mentioned a story we'd heard about a woman who was having her baby in the old maternity building at King's. She was using a birthing pool, tended by a sympathetic midwife, and everything was going well. Then there was a change of shift and a new midwife took over. This midwife disappeared for an hour 'to do her paperwork'. When she returned, she said that she couldn't measure the mother in the birthing pool and told her to get out. The mother was reluctant. So the midwife took away the gas and air and physically pulled the mother out of the birthing pool in the middle of a contraction. The mother ended up having a Caesarean.

The consultant midwife said that she was dealing with the 'serious allegations' I was referring to. Other pregnant couples said that they had heard similar stories about bullying or impatient members of staff. The consultant midwife was dismayed. I asked her what we could do in a situation like that. It's unlikely to happen, but it's possible. What are our rights if we are confronted by an unreasonable member of staff?

The consultant midwife said that nothing will be done without consultation with us. 'Staff will explain to you why they're doing what they're doing.'

In other words, they'll explain why they're right and you're wrong. It sounds fine in theory. But if there's still a disagreement about how to proceed with the labour, is the final decision ours or theirs? I still don't know the answer to this.

The consultant midwife eventually conceded that we 'might have to be assertive. If you don't say what you want, the staff might make assumptions. Often it's up to the birthing partner to be the assertive one.'

It's not an easy judgement to make. Tens of thousands of mothers and babies are helped by hospital staff every year; many of them owe their lives to doctors and midwives. But I know from experience that the quality of service in the NHS varies according to the skill, personality and mood of the person looking after you. Not many pregnant woman or birthing partners have the competence or the confidence to challenge the instructions or behaviour of medical personnel.

Maybe I'm overcompensating for this feeling of powerlessness. Probably everything will be fine.

Kate arrived from work. 'I haven't been feeling well the past couple of days,' she said. 'Heartburn. Farty. Tired.'

On the sofa she cuddled up to me. I could tell that she was about to tell me something that she thought I might not like. She said, 'Apparently, many women don't feel very sexual when they're breastfeeding. It's an evolutionary thing. If the woman doesn't have sex, she doesn't get pregnant again, so there's a plentiful supply of milk for the baby. I read it in the pink book.'

Age is a high price to pay for maturity, wrote Tom Stoppard. I would add to that. Celibacy is a high price to pay for children.

Now and again, I wobble. I think, why are we doing this, why am I doing this? Did I ever have rational reasons for wanting a baby? I've forgotten. I feel like I've been mugged by my genes. What was I thinking of?

Talking to the baby cheers me up.

Thursday 3 April

Kate's mum has come to visit. For five days. Kate wanted her mum to feel the baby move. The baby obliged by having hiccups.

Another present. *Un sac de nuit*. It's a sleeping bag with shoulder straps, a kind of padded dress longer than the baby and sealed with a zip at the bottom. It stops a baby slipping under the bedcovers and suffocating.

John phoned for advice. There's a woman he likes. But she won't be visiting London until next month. Should he suggest meeting up with her this weekend? He would have to drive to Leicester where she lives, a round trip of 300 miles. Or would that make him seem too keen? I told him to take the initiative, show that he's interested, seize the dame. If he waits six weeks and she's as gorgeous as he says she is, she might not be single then.

I'm trying to feel pleased for him. I am pleased for him. But part of me envies him the thrill of the chase.

Contentment doesn't mean living without ambivalence; it means learning to live with it. Even after you've made a commitment to someone, you're not entirely free of curiosity about your unlived lives. 'Weep for the lives your wishes never led,' said Auden. As I get older and make choices, it becomes increasingly unlikely that I'm ever going to play for England or fuck Kylie or fuck a black woman or have a threesome or drive to Leicester for sex; so I suffer from occasional bouts of lostalgia, a perverse form of nostalgia, a sense of yearning for things that have never happened, a sentimental longing for things that I'm never going to experience.

Kate has been feeling contractions in her belly.

Friday 4 April

Kate's mum came along to this morning's antenatal appointment at King's. In the waiting room, Kate kept saying, 'There!' and we looked at her belly, but always too late, we'd missed the movement. Then we stared for a minute, navel-gazing, but nothing happened. When we looked away, Kate shouted, 'There!' again.

It was Andrea, a midwife we've seen a couple of times. She felt the position of the baby's head. Kate asked if she could feel it as well, so Andrea showed her where to put her hands, at the bottom of the bump.

'Is the head meant to be that low?' asked Kate.

'It's not really low, you can move it from side to side, which shows it's not in the pelvis yet.' Our baby is lying on the right side. 'There's more of a bump there,' said Andrea. 'You're growing very nicely, anyway.'

Kate mentioned the contractions. The midwife said they're not contractions. 'It sounds like ligament pain. The broad ligaments supporting the uterus are very stretched.'

Amplified by the machine, the baby's heartbeat sounded like a galloping horse. One hundred and forty beats per minute. The baby's mum, dad and granny listened and smiled. We are an easy audience to please. All the baby has to do is breathe and we are delighted. 'It sounds good,' said the midwife.

All we want now is for the results of the MRI scan to confirm that there's nothing amiss with our baby's head. That's next Tuesday.

At the reception desk we made an appointment for our next antenatal check. Another Friday, three weeks away.

'Eleven o'clock?' asked the receptionist.

'I can only do nine o'clock,' said Kate.

'There's no space then. Oh well, come in at nine o'clock anyway. That's what I used to do.'

The staff were moaning about being understaffed. The receptionist, complaining that a member of staff had been summoned to the scanning room, said 'We need that like we need a hole in the head.' An unfortunate choice of phrase.

We walked home in sunny weather and sunny moods until Kate realised that she had left her bag in a toilet at the hospital. It contained her credit cards, her glasses, keys for the flat and keys for work.

We phoned the antenatal ward and they went to search the toilet. The bag wasn't there. Kate started to cry. 'I don't normally lose things,' she said. Her mum gave her a hug. I said that we should go home and I would cycle to the hospital and look for it myself. When we got home, there was a message from the antenatal ward. They had found the bag.

Saturday 5 April

We woke up early. 'Did you hear me groan in pain?' Kate asked.

'No.'

'I had a really sore knee. I couldn't move it. I hope I haven't got rheumatoid arthritis. Pregnancy can bring it on. My hips are really sore as well.'

I gave her a hug.

'You're squashing my breasts,' she said.

It's almost impossible to be in the same room as her without squashing her breasts.

Later, I phoned a friend. I'd been talking on the phone for less than five minutes.

'Are you still on the phone?' she said. 'We want to go.'

I ended my conversation prematurely and hung up the phone. Half an hour later, she still wasn't ready to leave the house.

She wanted me to spend the day with her and her mum. But as we were setting off and she was complaining about something else, I began to have second thoughts. I said that I might stay at home and work instead.

'I won't be grumpy all day,' she said. 'Come on. It's a sunny day.'

We went to the Active Birth Centre in Hampstead where I was encouraged to try on a Wilkinet, a type of baby carrier. It enables you to strap your baby to your chest or your back. The assistant gave me a doll to practise with. I began to thread and wrap long ribbons of material around my body. It's like trying to wrap a parcel when you're the parcel. All the women in the room – Kate, her mum, the shop assistant, other customers – stopped to watch the stupid man. Everything was going well until the last moment. I accidentally pulled the straps tight across the thighs, cutting off the blood supply to the doll's legs. All the women laughed.

It's not easy for a pregnant woman to find somewhere to pee on Hampstead Heath at this time of year. There aren't many leaves on the bushes. After a picnic, we strolled over Parliament Hill, dodging the kites. Kate said something. I kissed her. It was nearly 5 pm.

'Why do I deserve a kiss?'

'Because that's the first thing you've said all day that wasn't grumpy.'

We walked to a tube station. For Kate, the pregnancy is becoming a physical ordeal. A street feels like a mountain.

On the train Kate slept with her head on her mum's shoulder. When she woke up and stood up, she felt dizzy. After a drink of water, she said she felt well enough to continue walking.

We strolled along the Thames towpath from Putney Bridge to Hammersmith. Kate was weary. She emptied everything out of her pockets, even her tissues, and put them in my bag, to make herself lighter. This is my role. I am the mule.

We walked to St Paul's Church in Hammersmith to listen to Bach's mass in B minor. Our friend in the choir hasn't seen Kate for several months. Perhaps the excitement of performing made him less sensitive than he usually is. We chatted to him during the interval. It was the first thing he said to her: 'You've put on a lot of weight!'

Sunday 6 April   Week 34

Clare came round for tea and biscuits.

'Last night someone said I've put on a lot of weight,' Kate told her. 'But I haven't!' She laughed nervously. She was satirising herself, but she was also inviting our friend to say *that's right, you haven't put on a lot of weight*.

Our friend didn't say anything. She kept her thoughts to herself. She is in the position we used to be in: occasionally thinking about having kids, but not sure if it's worth it. If I remember correctly, childless people often console themselves by dwelling on the devastation inflicted on parents' bodies and social lives.

Kate is still reluctant to admit that pregnancy has rendered her mentally disadvantaged. Who am I to argue? I can only report, among other minor incidents, that we returned from the supermarket without tomatoes because she put them in somebody else's trolley.

Recklessly, we are daring to think about the future. Inspired by last night's concert, I suggested to Kate this morning that our child might want to learn how to play a musical instrument.

'Not the violin,' said Kate. 'It's hard to listen to, when someone's practising.'

Over supper, continuing the conversation, I said to Kate: 'We'll have to give Alice an instrument she can learn wearing headphones.'

Kate flinched in her seat as if she'd been electrocuted. And then I realised why she was so shocked. I had said the A word. I had spoken our baby's name, aloud, in public. I looked at Kate's mum, sitting at the table with us, a metre away. Head down, she wasn't listening anyway. She was preoccupied with peeling the skin off her trout. Had she heard? I don't know. I don't really care.

I've been feeling trapped and glum.

Unlike our grandparents' generation, people of our age weren't brought up with the expectation of squeezing our lives into rigid social and familial hierarchies. We were given more opportunities, greater hopes of self-determination and self-fulfilment. Having children has become a lifestyle choice rather than an obligation. The tension arises when people who are intellectually and temperamentally allergic to family life find themselves with a family of their own because of insidious and irresistible biological urges.

I'm not a reluctant dad. I can put up with less sleep and less sex. But if I have to give up writing, it'll be like losing a limb. Our baby's life is something to celebrate. I'm just worried about how much of my own life has to be subsumed and sacrificed.

Monday 7 April
I am boring myself with all this fretting and interior whining about lack of money and time. I need to snap out of it. I'm lucky to be having a baby.

This evening we went to our second Parent Education class. More people turned up this week. There were 21 of us. The midwife, Yvonne, looked tactlessly slim and sporty with purple nails and unsensible shoes. Again she provided an informative and entertaining two hours. This week she described the three stages of labour. Everything we could possibly want to know about mucus plugs and vaginal tearing.

We were divided into groups and given cards to stick on to a large sheet of paper. It felt like primary school. The cards described the typical symptoms experienced by women during birth. We had to attach each symptom to the appropriate stage of labour. The cards said things like 'My feet are freezing' and 'I really need to pee' and 'I feel confused'. Under the heading for the third stage of labour, my group attached a card saying 'I want to be alone' and another card saying 'Don't leave me alone'. Clearly we are already confused.

The first stage of labour is the dilation of the cervix from 0–10 centimetres. For first-time mothers, this first stage normally lasts for 10–12 hours. It's advisable to stay at home for as long as possible. 'You're more likely to have an intervention if you come into labour ward early,' said Yvonne.

Between the first and second stages, there is a transition stage. This can cause a dramatic change in behaviour. Quiet women start swearing loudly. Loud women might turn strangely quiet.

The second stage of labour is the baby's journey out of the womb. The woman will feel a strong urge to push when she's ready. She can't stop herself pushing. Pushing is involuntary.

Yvonne said, 'Your body is taking over now. You don't have any control over what's happening. The Hollywood movies are all wrong when they show midwives shouting "PUSH! PUSH!" I've never said to anybody to push. They know.'

She is full of useful tips. 'Bring a mirror. Why should you be the last person to see your baby?' Another useful tip: 'Don't scream. You can't scream and push at the same time. When you scream, all the energy is coming through your neck.'

The second stage might take half an hour or two hours. Yvonne says, 'It's not gonna fly out like Superman. It takes a while.'

At one point the baby might go into a vaginal dip and appear to be going backwards. Some women panic when they see this. 'IT'S GOING BACK-WARDS!' they scream.

The baby's presence causes rectal pressure, making the woman feel mistakenly that she needs to pooh. 'This is how babies are born on the toilet,' said Yvonne.

Getting the head out is the first challenge. The head is the hardest and largest part of the body. After that 'it's plain sailing … it may take one or two pushes to get the body out'.

Kate asked if rubbing wheatgerm oil into the perineum during labour would reduce the risk of tearing the perineum. Yvonne said, 'You can do it. I don't know if it's gonna do any good, but it won't do any harm.'

The third stage of labour is the delivery of the placenta. Some people like to take it home, fry it and eat it. We won't be doing that.

During the tea break we talked about water births to a woman called LIZZIE. She was concerned that the hospital has only two birthing pools, but the midwife assured her that there's always a pool available. According to LIZZIE, 'A lot of women think it's a good idea but chicken out when the pain starts and demand the drugs.'

For the last hour we were told about the four main options for pain relief. TENS. Entonox. Pethidine. Epidural.

Yvonne explained that we wouldn't be talking about breathing exercises. 'We don't do breathing in this class! What I would say about breathing is just do it. In seven years as a midwife I've never seen anyone do the breathing thing. Save your money!'

There isn't much good news. TENS stands for Transcutaneous Electrical Nerve Stimulation. Pads placed on the woman's back emit electrical pulses that supposedly stimulate the body's natural pain relievers. It might help. It might not. 'You've got nothing to lose,' Yvonne said. 'There are no side effects. It might enable you to stay at home for longer.' A TENS machine is used by 5.8 per cent of first-time mothers.

Entonox is a fancy term for gas and air. This is 50 per cent nitrous oxide and 50 per cent oxygen. It's similar to laughing gas. It can make you nauseous and light-headed. It usually has an effect within 40 seconds. It is used by 53.7 per cent of first-time mothers. Doctors and nurses use it at parties.

Pethidine is an opiate analgesic (a synthetic form of morphine) injected into thigh muscle. It takes effect within 15–20 minutes and lasts for 3 hours. It is used by 19.6 per cent of first-time mothers. It can make the mother feel sleepy or sick. It's not good for someone who wants to breastfeed. It can depress the baby's suck reflex. Yvonne says it only works in 20 per cent of cases. 'People who come to Parent Classes tend to say no to pethidine.'

TRACY asked, 'Why do some people still take it when there are so many potential side effects?'

Yvonne said, 'It's difficult to get through to someone when they're screaming.'

An epidural takes effect within 20–30 minutes. It increases the chances of an intervention. It causes a persistent headache in 1 per cent of women as a result of losing cerebrospinal fluid. It can lower the mother's blood pressure. It is used by 44.6 per cent of first-time mothers. That figure includes women who have Caesareans, or 'caesars' as they are sometimes called.

Ten point six per cent of women use no pain relief.

These statistics come from King's, where 4,000 babies are born every year.

LIZZIE said a friend of hers used a *doula*. This is a Greek word meaning 'wise woman'. Basically it's a professional birthing partner who provides extra support during the labour. I'd never heard of this word before. Neither had GARY. He said earnestly, 'A what? A dealer?' He thought it was another source of drugs.

'We want to hear your baby cry once it's out,' said Yvonne. 'We don't hit babies any more. When it comes out we just rub it with an NHS towel and that usually does the trick.'

There's one more class next week. After that, Kate has also booked us for six classes organised by the National Childbirth Trust, each one lasting two hours.

'It's hard work, eh?' said Kate's mum.

'Yeah,' I agreed, 'We'll be exhausted by the time the baby gets here.'

When Susanne was pregnant with Kate in 1969, there were no scans, no dietary recommendations and no antenatal classes.

Tuesday 8 April
I've been dreading today. And I've been impatient for it to arrive.

Kate's mum came with us to the hospital. For yet another ultrasound scan. And to hear the results of the MRI scan. So we'll know if there is any bleeding or abnormal development inside our baby's brain.

The woman was friendly. 'I'm Tina.' She invited us into the scanning room. There was a crowd of students in there. Kate said to Tina, 'Last time there were eight people and I'd like fewer people this time.' The crowd left. Only Tina stayed behind, to operate the scanner, and a man and a woman who whispered over the computer as they entered the data.

We were told that they hadn't received the MRI results yet. Kate explained that the MRI scan was ten days ago and we had come today for the results. Tina said that they would try to find them. The other woman said the problem was that 'the midwife is off sick'.

Once again we watched the shapes and shadows of our baby's brain on the monitor as the measurements were taken. The ventricle was about the same size as last time. This is good news. It is stable. It isn't progressive enlargement.

While we waited for the consultant to arrive, we were given a tour of our baby. The machine's narrow angle of view meant that we couldn't see an overall picture of the baby in the womb. Instead, individual components became recognisable. A hand. A foot. The spine. An eye.

'Oh look!' said Tina, excited. On the screen we saw the top of the spine. The nape of the neck. And the back of the skull covered in white flames. Tina explained, 'It's hair!' A narrow ridge of it over the skull. Our baby has a Mohican. 'She's a hairy little thing!' said Tina. We expected this. The baby's mum and dad are quite hairy.

Then Tina was replaced by another woman. This was the fourth different consultant we've met over these weeks of scanning. She didn't introduce herself, didn't look at Kate, didn't make eye contact. Later we saw on the report that her name was Deborah.

Of all the senior consultants we've spoken to, she had the most reassuring opinion about the scan results. She seemed unconcerned, almost unimpressed, by the size of the baby's ventricles. 'It's likely to be a normal variant,' she told us after checking the measurements, 'in 95 per cent of cases this will be a normal baby.'

(Kate said afterwards, 'Did you see her face when she saw the ventricle measurements? She looked as if she thought too much fuss had been made and we'd been put through this unnecessarily. But who knows? Maybe I'm overinterpreting.')

We still hadn't received the results of the MRI scan. The consultant said that, if they failed to obtain them today, they would send them to us in the post. Kate said that we would prefer to know today. 'We don't mind waiting.'

So we waited. After 20 minutes the consultant called us into another room. She had the MRI results. She said, 'It confirms what we already know. There is a slight prominence of the ventricles. But that's all. Some-times there is a structure in the brain that is also missing, but that structure is clearly visible on your baby's scan. There is no cerebral malformation.'

'So … do we need any more scans?'

'No.'

'I feel like celebrating,' said Kate outside the hospital, 'with a cake.' In the absence of cake, we celebrated with a kiss.

I phoned my mum to tell her the good news because I knew she'd be worrying. I could hear the relief in her voice. She said, 'I thought you were getting the results on Thursday. I don't know why I thought that.'

I met a neighbour in the street. I told her about the baby. 'You know how they measure everything? At the second scan there was one measurement that was slightly outside the normal range. So we've had five scans. And this morning we got the final results. It's fine.'

'So you're happy?'

I smiled and nodded. She smiled and said, 'Congratulations.'

I've been dreading today. It has turned out OK.

Wednesday 9 April

I woke up with an involuntary erection. I apologised to Kate as we cuddled like spoons. 'If you feel any rectal pressure, it's not the baby trying to get out, it's me trying to get in.'

'I'm sorry,' she said.

'Don't be sorry. Don't worry about it.' I've got used to it.

She decided that today we could begin perineal massage. Rubbing wheatgerm oil into the perineum four to six weeks before birth is supposed to improve the elasticity of the skin, reducing the chances of tearing. The oil can be self-applied or your partner can do it. One of the advantages of letting your partner do it, according to the leaflet we picked up at the Active Birth Centre, is that 'it can help to develop the cooperation, use of feedback and touch that you will need in labour'.

I cut my fingernails and washed my hands. Kate reclined on the bed, propped up by pillows, and I began to apply the wheatgerm oil with two fingers. I am supposed to insert my fingers 1–2 inches into the vaginal opening and pull the skin gently down towards the back passage and out (as the baby's head will do).

Kate was supposed to be relaxed. The leaflet mentioned this several times. *You must be relaxed for this to work.* In fact she was scowling and she kicked the duvet violently out of the way. Her tone of voice didn't sound relaxed as she gave me instructions. She seemed to blame me for being unable to find her anus. She sounded tetchy, but I had to remind myself that a degree of tetchiness wasn't unreasonable. *'You should feel a slight tingling or burning sensation, but not pain,'* said the leaflet.

We discussed how Kate will cope with the pain of labour if she doesn't take any powerful drugs. Although she has never experienced severe pain, she said, she has been 'on long hikes' where it was an ordeal to put one foot in front of the other. And that gives her hope. She hasn't got any experience to prove it, she said, but she's hopeful that she has enough strength of character to enable her to cope with the pain of giving birth. She thought for a moment. Then she said, 'Oh God.'

In a supermarket in Peckham, I saw a baby girl tucked into her pram, bright blue eyes peering at me as if I were an interesting alien. For the first time in weeks I allowed myself to really believe that soon we might be sharing our lives with such a cute and curious little baby. I was surprised by how happy this made me feel. From this new perspective, my recent doubts about the advisability of having a baby seemed obscene and ignorant.

In the next aisle I heard the shuffling feet of a boy of about 13 with Down's syndrome. He was being dragged along by his grim-faced mother.

Parents are dependent on their children. The health and personality of our child will largely determine how we live the rest of our lives.

Thursday 10 April
I phoned Kate at work. 'How are you?'

'Really tired and farty.' She sounded half-asleep.

I went to the supermarket and forgot to buy the thing I'd gone there for. I'm always like this when I'm working. Writing is a form of dementia. The gap between the imaginative world and the real world is too great for an immediate transition. It's not like flicking a switch. It's like coming to the surface from the bottom of the sea. I'm not absent-minded. I'm present-minded elsewhere. I'm concerned that this will make me a liability as a parent, and I will screw up all the simple routines of childcare. I'm worried that I'll leave the baby in a shop.

It happens. My friend once left his baby sitting in a car seat on the pavement. It remained there for half an hour until a neighbour noticed. I've heard of another dad who has a habit of driving to the supermarket, parking the car and forgetting to take the baby inside with him.

I feel in a rush all the time. There's so much work I want to do while I still can. Kate is similarly possessed. She said that she would be home by 6.30 pm. I phoned her at 7 pm. She was still at the office. 'I'm sorry.' She sounded exhausted.

Our baby will need about 4,500 nappy changes in 2½ years; 4½ trees are destroyed to keep one baby in disposable nappies for 30 months; it takes a cupful of crude oil to produce the plastic for one disposable nappy; a disposable nappy takes 200 to 500 years to decompose; nappies will comprise 50 per cent of our household waste. Eight million disposable nappies are used in the UK every day. They comprise 4 per cent of the nation's household waste. In one year, a baby uses enough nappies to cover half a football pitch.

We're comparing the options. A newborn baby requires six to ten nappies per day. Let's say eight per day. That's 2,920 nappies per year. Costing £554.80 for biodegradable Tushies or £312.44 for indestructible Huggies.

We've not keen on the idea of washable nappies because a) this is a small flat and we don't want to be tripping over damp nappies and b) we don't want to devote all that time to rinsing and washing and drying. Apparently there's a company that will take away your dirty nappies and replace them with cleaned ones. So we'll have to look into that. When I get a second, I'll add it to my list of things to do. One of the things on my list of things to do is to look at my list of things to do.

Kate phoned a friend. 'It's starting to feel really close now. It's a bit scary.' She saw her reflection in the window. 'I'm huge!'

Friday 11 April

Ollie said, 'If we can't get the film made with Tim Roth and Rachel Weisz attached, we don't deserve to call ourselves producers.' That was five years ago. He failed. Now he's trying again. He is persistent, if nothing else. His heart is in the right place; but his brain goes AWOL now and again. He has just returned from Los Angeles. I phoned, wondering what progress he's made. He says that our executive producer, Edward, is 'a twisted bastard and I wouldn't trust him further than I can throw him'. I'm not hopeful.

Took a train from Waterloo to Brockenhurst, near the New Forest.

We're staying with friends who live in Lymington, a pretty town on the edge of the mainland, across from the Isle of Wight. We spent the evening talking about pregnancy, birth and babies. What did we used to talk about? I've forgotten. Nothing else is so interesting.

When she was admitted to hospital for her second child to be born, Carol was waiting on the labour ward, listening to the conversation in the next bed. A young male nurse asked the woman, 'How do you feel about being induced now?'

The woman was shocked. 'But I'm only twenty-five weeks pregnant.'

'Oh,' said the male nurse. 'Are you Carol Henman?'

'No!'

'I'm over here,' said Carol from the next bed.

Carol gives us hope that the birth might not be quite as bad as we fear. She had so much gas and air that she felt as if she was watching the birth from the ceiling. 'It's painful but it's not arrrggggghh painful. It's just absolutely exhausting.'

Saturday 12 April

Kate was restless. She needed more pillows. She wanted me further away. She wanted me closer. She fell asleep at last and I lay with my arm around her belly.

The baby woke at six. I could feel the seismic tremors. Like she was trying to fight her way out. I felt a surge of love for the baby. This love is like a tidal river, with high and low tides, but constantly flowing, and mingled with sewage and household waste and various detritus from other places.

Eventually light seeped into the room. Outside there was a choir of quacking, cooing, chirping and tweeting. The whole repertoire. Just before seven o'clock there was a squawk from inside the house. 'Mummy!'

The day had begun.

Our friends have two lovable daughters aged five and three. For us, today was an insight into the realities of parenthood, to which we've committed the rest of our lives despite our complete lack of personal experience. Today was a kind of belated test drive.

I'd played six games of noughts and crosses and a game of snakes and ladders before I'd even got out of bed. Betty, the eldest, is bright and sweet-natured, inexhaustible and exhausting, constantly doing cartwheels and handstands and 'rolypolys' (a forward roll). After breakfast I made a swan and a dog out of balloons.

We all took a boat to Hurst Castle, a fortification on a spit of shingle opposite the Needles. Betty collected shells and she was delighted when we found a set of false teeth on the beach. On the boat back to Lymington, we did sums and played I Spy. By late afternoon I had come to appreciate the simple parental pleasure of just sitting down.

In the evening, stories. I read *My Naughty Little Sister* to Betty. Then the kids went to sleep, and the adults shared another simple parental pleasure. A video. *The Shipping News*. Our friends made a special effort for us and stayed awake. They often rent videos but rarely get to the end.

Sunday 13 April   Week 35

A day with kids ensured that we slept solidly. Woke up at 9 am. Eddie, also a football addict, was keen to watch the highlights on ITV, but Betty was watching a video of *The Neverending Story*. Luckily her concentration wasn't never-ending and we managed to see the last 20 minutes of the football. But the enjoyment wasn't the same, knowing that there were kids wanting attention. The time spent watching television felt like something naughty, stolen from children.

I listen to other parents to prepare myself for what's to come. But they rarely seem to agree. I've been told that the first three months are a whirlwind and then things calm down. Eddie tells me the opposite. The first three months give you a false optimism, he says. The baby just sleeps and you can get on with other things.

Carol asked us, 'What equipment have you got?' This made us feel uneasy. We haven't got anything yet. I remember one of the books asking 'What clothes have you bought your baby?' That was at the end of week 25.

In the afternoon Eddie and I went to the pub to watch Southampton win the FA Cup semi-final. Carol took the kids to a children's party. Kate stayed at home to rest and read, and to avoid the children's party. She felt painful spasms in her abdomen, strong enough to make her scared that she was going into labour. She realised that she didn't know where anyone was. Her mobile had a flat battery and she didn't have my mobile number in her head. Her medical notes, which we were told to carry everywhere, are a hundred miles away in Peckham.

Kate can't stand still. She sways from side to side to alleviate the pain in her hip. The discomforts are multiplying. 'I haven't poohed for two days,' she told me later.

We were playing in the garden with the kids. Carol came out to put washing on the line. She hasn't been to our flat in London. She said, 'Have you got a garden?'

'No,' said Kate. 'But we're going to get a heated towel rail.'

I can see the benefits of life in a small town. The kids have a bedroom each, a garden, a conservatory. The house is left unlocked when the family goes for a walk to the harbour. They see deer in the lane.

And then our train was arriving at Waterloo station and I felt the excitement of London again. We don't have deer in Peckham. But we have foxes in the street.

Our last meal with our friends was an Indian takeaway. Kate was awake half the night, vomiting.

Monday 14 April

Kate took the day off work, something she never does. 'I can still smell vomit up my nose.' I cooked her lunch. A bowl of plain rice.

We made lists of things we need. Baby clothes. Baby equipment. Things to take to the hospital. Just writing it all down took a couple of hours.

In the newspapers I see articles calculating the cost of a child over 18 years. It's about £300,000. I've never had much disposable income. Now I have none. I have disposed income.

The rest of the afternoon was full of chores. Washing clothes. Putting the bin out. Vacuuming, because Kate said the dust in the bedroom was making her cough. I thought about all the writing I should be doing. Exasperated, I groaned out loud. Kate heard me. She said, 'What?'

'Nothing,' I said. 'I'm just feeling trapped.'

'By what?'

'By my life.'

Not the most sensitive thing I've ever said. I probably shouldn't have mentioned it. A problem shared is a problem doubled. Sometimes it's good to talk; sometimes you should just keep your mouth shut.

Kate has also been feeling exasperated by life. She told me that one day last week, on her way home from work, she was surprised when her bus terminated at Herne Hill. She asked the bus driver for her ticket back, so she could complete her journey. He refused. She got off the bus and burst into tears. She felt a surge of anger. She almost kicked the door as she disembarked. The bus driver pointed to the sign on the front of the bus saying HERNE HILL. Kate stuck up her middle finger.

Only 12 people turned up for the antenatal class at Dulwich Hospital. Perhaps people were deterred by the topic. Tonight we were talking about what happens if things go wrong.

We were divided into three groups and invited to write down questions about induction, instrumental delivery and Caesarean.

In this country, if a woman hasn't given birth after 42 weeks, the baby is induced while the placenta is still strong enough to withstand the rigours of labour. One or two milligrams of prostin are injected into the vagina, behind the cervix, and left for six hours. Then your membranes are ruptured with a small hook that looks like a knitting needle. The moment of rupture isn't painful, but getting to the membrane can be painful. It depends on the talent of the person using the hook.

It's not really known why some women don't go into labour naturally. 'Before I came into this profession, I thought doctors knew everything,' said Yvonne. 'But they don't. There's a lot they don't know.'

Someone asked if labour can be induced 'by shagging or having a beef vindaloo'. Yvonne said it's worth a try. Sperm also contains prostaglandin. 'Obviously there's more of it in the injected gel. Well, I don't know. I don't want to cast aspersions.'

An assisted delivery using instruments such as forceps or a ventouse occurs if the second stage of labour is prolonged. Otherwise the baby's head might get squashed or its heart rate might go down. After one and a half hours of pushing, the baby should be out. If it isn't, the doctors might help it along with a ventouse, a kind of suction cap attached to the baby's head. Yvonne showed us a metal one, like an old bath plug attached to a hollow rubber tube.

After three pulls with a ventouse, if the baby is still reluctant to come out, they resort to the forceps. A pair was passed around the room, clanking together awkwardly in our clumsy hands.

Someone asked, 'How hard do they pull?'

Yvonne said, 'It looks harder than it is. I can't really answer that because I don't use them.' In her career, she has encountered one delivery with a ventouse and none with forceps. Nationally the ventouse rate is 5 per cent and the forceps rate is 3 per cent. Yvonne says we can reduce the chances of an intervention by staying at home as long as possible.

If three tugs with the forceps don't bring the baby out, the doctors will recommend a Caesarean. This is also suggested if there are signs that the baby is distressed. Twenty-five per cent of births at King's are Caesareans, although half of those are prearranged.

Ideally the Caesarean is performed using an epidural rather than a general anaesthetic. If a general anaesthetic is required, Yvonne explained, it can be difficult putting a tube down the unconscious mother's engorged throat. As she spoke, some of the pregnant women were looking uneasy.

My small group had written a list of questions about Caesareans. I had to read them out. 'Is a Caesarean always necessary, or are doctors sometimes impatient or lazy?'

Yvonne, trying to be diplomatic but honest, said, 'If I was having a baby, there are some obstetricians I'd prefer to have around and some I'd prefer to avoid.'

Some women seemed troubled by all these bleak possibilities. One of them in particular. She was a large woman who was normally chatty and cheerful. At the start of the meeting she had announced, 'I had a magic moment last night. I was slumped in front of the telly and I found that I could rest my cup of tea on my bump.' Now she wasn't so jolly. She seemed scared. 'Can we talk about post-natal stuff?' she said. 'That's what I want to know about.' So we moved on.

We were divided into two quiz teams. People were remarkably competitive – to the point of insensitivity. My team was heckled while we tried to think of five ways to avoid cot death. This was worth ten points. 'Don't let the baby smoke?' suggested one man.

What can the partner do to help in the days after birth?

'Keeping people away,' said Yvonne, 'is one very important job the partner has. Change your answerphone message.'

She suggests something along these lines: 'Hello, thank you for calling. Our baby is a little girl, born on Friday the seventh at 9 o'clock in the evening, she weighed 7 pounds 10 ounces, her name is Jemima. Leave your name and number and we'll call you back in six months.'

Tuesday 15 April

Kate felt better today and went to work. I ignored the sunshine and stayed indoors, tapping at the computer, enjoying an uninterrupted day of work while I still can.

In the evening I cycled into central London. The sun was a cause of near nudity on the streets of Soho. I met John. We sat on the grass in Soho Square among a crowd of summery people. We ate Thai food and watched a peculiar Spanish movie, *Intacto*, reminiscent of Roald Dahl's stories.

John is healthy, successful in his career, affluent, liked, respected … and unhappy. Because he can't find a girlfriend. Not one that he really likes, anyway. There are moments when it's tempting to look back on single life as an enchanted time of carefree hedonism. It's helpful to have miserable single friends.

I got home at midnight. In bed I said, 'Are you OK, lovey?'

'No.'

'What's up?'

'Burning.'

There was a fire raging in the middle of her chest. She took some Mucogel. The good news is that it doesn't taste as bad as it sounds. The bad news is that it doesn't work. It has no side effects – but it has no effects, either.

Wednesday 16 April

Kate is finding it difficult to follow all the advice she has been given. She is supposed to sit with her feet up. She is also supposed to sit forward to ease the heartburn. It's not particularly easy to sit forward when you've got your feet up, especially when you've got a big bump in the middle.

I brought her sandals down from the loft. A sign of summer. Also a sign that her feet have swollen and she can't fit into her shoes. She is starting to look like a balloon animal.

Kate met a friend for lunch. Walking home afterwards, she looked down and was overwhelmed. 'I thought, how weird, how bizarre, that I have this big bump. And inside is a baby with a brain and a nose and eyes.'

I have the same feeling sometimes when I look at her. How strange the whole process is. How animalistic. How physical and fleshy and messy. Her body is no longer a single-occupant dwelling. A woman's body is adorned and adored, cherished and caressed, massaged and moisturised, exercised and exfoliated, publicly displayed but only visited by private invitation. And suddenly it is invaded, usurped. There is a squatter, a lodger, a housemate.

On the south bank of the Thames is Tate Modern, an art gallery converted from an old power station. It has been a successful and popular transformation. Now people regard the old industrial chimney and the cavernous turbine hall as aesthetic objects. They don't just revere the works of art but also the building that contains them. Kate's body has undergone the opposite conversion. It has turned into something utilitarian, and we are seeing that many of her most aesthetic components are primarily functional. The pleasure palace has been turned into a factory.

Thursday 17 April

More sunshine. I went for a meandering bike ride and ended up at Nunhead Cemetery.

Saw a headstone 'to commemorate the scouts of the 2nd Walworth troop drowned off Leysdown, Isle of Sheppey, on 4th August 1912'. There were 9 names of children aged 11–14, including 2 from the same family, Noel Filmer aged 14 and Thompson Filmer aged 12. Behind this memorial stone lay five rows of graves for New Zealanders killed in the First World War. Some of these soldiers were only 18 years old. One of them had an inscription:

> HOW MANY HOPES
> LIE BURIED HERE
> MOTHER

Many of the graves are family vaults from the 19th century, their inscriptions hinting at histories as complicated and tragic as a Victorian novel.

Proximity to so many dead people with varying fates, so many lost lives and forgotten tragedies, slowed me down, stilled my simmering mind, stopped me obsessing about things that aren't worth worrying about. This wiser perspective lasted until I got home and realised how much work I have to do.

Kate phoned as she was leaving work and suggested that we could meet in Brockwell Park. I met her by the lido. The prospect of ice cream motivated her to climb the hill to the café. We sat on the grass among the sunbathers and watched her stomach twitching.

'I had a dream last night,' she said. 'I gave birth and you weren't there.'

'I promise you, lovey, I will be there.'

'And the baby was born without a head. In the world of the dream, that was normal. The head was supposed to grow later. But I was worried that its head wasn't growing properly.'

'I promise you our baby will be born with a head.'

Kate keeps being surprised by herself. 'I feel heavy today … I'm huge … I can't move like I used to move … I'm a heffalump … I'm definitely huge now. Isn't that amazing? There's a baby in there.'

Friday 18 April

Half-asleep, getting out of bed to go for a pee in the early hours, Kate was struggling to get upright. I was woken by the tremors in the mattress as she strained to move. 'Are you all right?'

'Give me a push,' she said.

One shove and she was up and free again.

She didn't sleep well. Mysterious pains in her left hip and left knee kept her awake.

Our friend, who had an early miscarriage a few months ago, has written to say that she is pregnant again.

In a local newspaper a while ago I read about a cyclist who was transporting long poles on his bike, strapped across the handlebars. At a roundabout, weaving between vehicles, the cyclist fell off and was killed by a lorry. The dead cyclist was a Road Safety Officer for the local council.

I remembered this story today when I was cycling home from the supermarket with a carrier bag of shopping dangling from my handlebars. I had hoped, now that we're having a baby, that a sense of responsibility would make me less stupid. This new maturity hasn't manifested itself yet. I am still a dickhead.

We don't like the old pram that a friend has given us. It's so big that it blocks the hall. Tonight I tried to fold it up. It is supposed to be collapsible. We pushed and pulled the plastic knobs and levers, pressed against the heavy metal frame, and after half an hour we got it to collapse.

We looked in the baby equipment catalogues. Modern prams are called 'travel systems'. They have patterns with names like 'urban cool'. Some of them cost £450.

My producer claims that he still can't afford to pay me for any of the unpaid rewrites. He described his financial situation as 'desperate'. Then he said that he is going to be away for a few days. When I pressed him, he said he is taking his family to the South of France.

Saturday 19 April

My gran has been moved to a hospital ward for stroke victims. She has a faulty inner ear and she has trouble balancing. She is supposed to be confined to bed but yesterday she was taken to the toilet by mistake. She vomited. Her speech and mobility have deteriorated so I can't speak to her on the phone. I've sent her a card. After her two previous strokes, she recovered her speech and got some of her strength back. We're hoping she will prove equally resilient this time as well. But nobody knows what's going to happen, even the doctors. The end of life is as unpredictable as the beginning. The hospital is on Lovely Lane, but it's not a lovely place. I hope she isn't too frightened in there. I hope Nana gets to meet my daughter. I hope my daughter gets to meet her great-grandmother.

So I can't moan, really, about my own petty frustrations. We have a habit of moaning because our glass is one-tenth empty.

Kate hardly ever grumbled before she was pregnant. Now she can be a bit cantankerous. I keep thinking I've done something to upset her. Today I said, 'Are you a bit crabby, lovey?'

'A little bit. I've got a headache and I'm hot and my belly's a bit sore.'

She is taking things easy while she is tired. 'I'm bored,' she said this morning. I suspect that's something she'll have to get used to. Kathy has given her advice about breastfeeding. 'Make sure the phone is within reach. It can be quite dull.'

Doris Lessing wrote: 'There is no boredom like that of an intelligent young woman who spends all day with a very small child.'

Kate says she is becoming impatient now. She is getting prepared. The washing machine was on all day.

Sunday 20 April   **Week 36**

Kate's waist has a circumference of 104½ centimetres (41½ inches). She has to suck her belly in when she zips and unzips her coat. Her maternity trousers fit her when she's standing up, but she has to undo the top button when she sits down.

'Is my bum bigger?' she asked me.

In relationships, there is no Fifth Amendment. You are obliged to incriminate yourself or perjure yourself. I chose perjury.

'No.'

Not that my own backside is exactly shrinking. I'm on the second notch of my belt. I blame the pregnancy. We have a less mobile, less active life. Less cycling, less walking, less sex. Same amount of cake.

Normally on a long weekend we would seek out a mountain and have a picnic on top of it. Today we settled for lunch in a pub opposite Peckham Rye. We walked, as ever, at a funereal pace.

We looked at photos from three years ago. Cycling on the South Downs. Hiking in the Italian Alps. 'How young we looked then,' said Kate. 'All the blotchiness on my skin makes me feel old.' She means the brown smudges that have appeared on her face over recent months. Pregnancy hormones can change the pigmentation of the skin. 'I hope it goes away afterwards.'

'I'm sure it will.' I have no idea if it will.

I looked it up. The books say that the brown splodges are caused by increased levels of melanocyte stimulating hormone (MSH), also responsible for the *linea nigra* and the darkening of the nipples and areolae. The irregular brown blotches are made worse by sunlight but 'usually begin to fade shortly after delivery and may disappear completely in a few months'.

'Sometimes it's overwhelming,' she says, 'this feeling that there's a baby inside me. I can't describe it. I feel as if, when she's out, it won't be so overwhelming.'

She is washing everything. Even the shower curtain. I have run out of places to hang things.

We've been given quite a few baby clothes, of various sizes. Kate has washed them and stacked them, the smallest one on top. The romper suits could fit inside each other like Russian dolls.

Monday 21 April

Everyone has an opinion. We went to a friend's picnic in Hyde Park, near the Serpentine. One mother told us that we're fortunate to be having a girl because girls are less aggressive than boys, even in the womb. Kate confirmed, happily, that our baby is 'a pusher not a kicker'.

We left the picnickers and went to visit Mothercare on Oxford Street. We bought a few small items that amounted to £44.

Then we went to Marks & Spencer. Kate was looking for a bathrobe to wear on the labour ward. She emerged instead with a purple denim jacket.

Babies, like dogs, allow people to talk to each other. A woman started chatting to us in Marks & Spencer. She saw Kate's belly and declared confidently, 'It's gonna be a boy. Girls lie top to bottom, boys lie side to side. That's definitely a boy.' She is the third person to say this. And it's true that, recently, the bump has become wider. The woman looked deflated when we told her that it was a girl.

It was after midnight. I'd just watched football on the telly. I turned on my computer to do some work. Kate had gone to bed an hour and a half earlier. Now she came into the room complaining of breathlessness, and asked me to take her pulse. She felt as if it was racing. I found a clock with a second hand. Her pulse was a regular 60 beats per minute. I told her it was normal. This is where the books can be useful, providing credible reassurance. I read out a section. It said that breathlessness is often a problem in late pregnancy when you have a lot of extra weight to carry around and lung space is restricted. One book recommended deep breathing, concentrating on breathing out and emptying the lungs. We did that for a couple of minutes. Calmer, she went back to bed.

You can't escape. But you can cope.

'Pregnant, I was my own prison,' wrote Lorna Sage in her autobiography. In the final months, a pregnant woman is sentenced to hard labour, subjected to varied and prolonged physical torments, saturated with chemicals that alter her mental and emotional state and deprived of sleep. Normally, when people suffer like this, it would be regarded as an abuse of human rights.

Tuesday 22 April

I phoned a friend I haven't spoken to since week 12.

'Are you a dad yet?'

'No, not for five weeks or so.'

'God, it takes so long, doesn't it.'

'Oh. It feels to us as if the time has passed quickly.'

I sense that I'm running out of days but I still waste half of them. If I had any sense, I would throw a brick at my television. I turn it on to watch the news and find myself watching cheap quiz shows. I am hypnotised by programmes from the 1970s. I am arrested and detained by *Starsky and Hutch*.

Choosing a pram turns out to be as complicated as choosing a car. Kate saw a woman getting off a bus holding a baby in one arm and a buggy in the other. Impressed by the compactness of the buggy, she asked the woman about it. It was a TRAX. It had cost £60 at a NCT nearly new sale. Nearly new is a middle-class way of saying second-hand.

Kate arrived home from work and started cleaning and dusting with a fervour I have never seen before. I can only conclude that, just as there are hormones that make a woman go into labour and lactate, there are also hormones that make her dust.

Another friend asked me the same question this evening. 'Are you a dad yet?' Clearly they haven't marked this momentous occasion in their calendar. To the rest of the world this is a mundane event.

If the world isn't particularly interested in us, the indifference is mutual. The world's tragedies were chronicled on *Newsnight*, but Kate wasn't looking. She was browsing through the Mothercare catalogue.

Wednesday 23 April
Ian and Jacqui's first pregnancy ended with an early miscarriage. Six months ago, during their second pregnancy, the ultrasound scan revealed an ovarian cyst. In this morning's mail, I received a photo of a baby chewing a blanket. This is their little boy, Jake, born on 28 March at 3.38 am weighing 6 pounds 10 ounces. His dad writes: 'It *is* definitely worth it – even Jacqui thinks so and she did much more of the hard stuff. Nothing prepares you for the worry though – or the overwhelming love.'

I keep thinking this: my mum went through pregnancy and parenthood on her own. She gave me a loving home, even though her own childhood had been violent. Today on the phone, I mentioned this. She said, 'I know what childhood can do to a person. I think mine made me a better parent. It made me stand up and decide that wasn't going to happen to my child.'

I said that I was grateful for what she'd done for me.

She said, 'You don't owe me nothing. What I did for you I did because I loved you. And you'll do the same for your baby.'

There's an organic vegetable shop on Northcross Road. Kate walked there and bought what she wanted. Then she phoned me and I cycled over and carried the bags home.

My gran often speaks with rose-tinted fondness of the old days when people sat in the street peeling their spuds and chatting. There is one community where a similar spirit of mutuality still exists – the pregnant community. Having a baby entitles you to membership of this secret society where there is free exchange of information and property. People are being very generous. A friend came round with his twins and left us some baby clothes and a TOMY baby carrier.

Thursday 24 April

We are public property. People ask me if the baby has been born yet. They wish me luck. How's Kate? How's her blood pressure? Are her feet swollen? Has she stopped work yet? Pregnancy is a minor form of celebrity. Andy Warhol was wrong. Everyone is famous for nine months. Then we become mere extras, and the baby is the star.

Kate got stuck on the sofa tonight.

I'm waiting for her to become intensely irritable and impatient, like the books say, but it hasn't happened yet. She hardly complains. As long as the baby is moving regularly, she's happy. I would be moaning a lot more.

Friday 25 April

We waddled over the hill to the hospital for an antenatal appointment. In the women's outpatients' department, menopausal women share a waiting room with pregnant women.

The midwife was a likeable, funny, rotund West Indian woman. 'My name's Mildred. I'm not permanent. They just call me when they're short, which they did last night at 11 o'clock. Is baby moving all right?'

'Yes,' said Kate.

'You got urine for me?'

'Yes.'

'You got any questions?'

Kate asked about Floradix, an iron supplement to combat fatigue. Is it OK to take it when you're breastfeeding? She feels energetic now but she thinks that this might change after the birth.

Mildred is a fan of Floradix. 'It's very nice, I think. I think they put rum in it. I take it every day in liquid form.'

Everyone else has said that liquid Floradix tastes disgusting. We weren't sure if Mildred was telling us a white lie. She suggested that Kate should start taking it, in liquid or tablet form, two weeks before the birth so that she builds up her reserves.

She measured Kate's blood pressure: 110 over 60. 'Not bad,' said Mildred. Kate lay down and Mildred felt the bump.

'The head hasn't engaged yet.'

'How can you tell?'

'I can feel it moving. You can feel it, too.' Mildred invited her to feel the baby's head. Kate didn't really want to.

'I can't,' said Kate. 'I can never really feel it.'

'You can, look, here.'

Mildred guided Kate's hands. 'Oh yes!' said Kate. (But she told me later that she was just pretending that she could feel it. She was too scared to press firmly.)

'Do you want to feel it?' Mildred asked me.

I really could feel the head, hard like an apple hidden under bulky clothing.

Then we listened to the heartbeat. It sounded like a drumbeat. My foot tapped along.

Mildred measured the bump from top to bottom with a tape measure. She said, 'Do you know why I'm doing this?'

'Yes,' said Kate. 'To measure the rate of growth.'

'And do you know what it's meant to be?'

'It's meant to grow two centimetres every two weeks.'

'Yes, one centimetre a week.'

The bump was 32 centimetres long. Mildred compared this to the last measurement taken a fortnight ago. That was also 32 centimetres long. 'It does not mean anything,' said Mildred. 'The baby might just be lazy today and curled up. They say that by week 35 the measurement should be 35 centimetres, but that is not always the case. You are not a big fat person.' She pointed to me. 'That is not a big person.' I sat up straighter in my chair.

We shared Mildred's lack of anxiety about the measurements. We have learnt to doubt their exactness and significance.

Later I was queuing at the till in Sainsbury's. A woman with two young children was behind me. Her trolley was stacked high with nappies and baby food. I said to her, 'I'm about to have a baby. It's frightening seeing how much you have to buy.'

'You get into the rhythm of it,' she said. 'Just forget about your past life completely.'

There was another woman in the queue. It was the comedienne Jo Brand, holding a blotchy-faced baby. Amid the demands of motherhood, she had still found time to paint her toenails red. This gives me hope. I can use the toenail-painting time for other things.

A man has delivered our new car. A blue Renault Scenic. Now we are polluters and congesters again. It rained heavily in the afternoon. I was pleased. I drove to Kate's work to give her a lift home, saving her from the rain, a knight in shining blue armour.

We went to Forest Hill to visit a friend, Sally, who gave us a car seat (and also a few toys and rattles and a large furry dog).

As we chatted, her daughter was happily scampering around the room. 'It's amazing. She starts out as a tiny thing that just screams and sucks, and 19 months later it's a little person running around. It's phenomenal.'

Not that the information we receive is always encouraging. This friend did not find breastfeeding to be a fulfilling experience. 'It was absolute bloody hell to be honest. And it's exhausting.'

'Did you take Floradix?' asked Kate.

'I did. I was still knackered.'

Kate was worrying, after all, about the measurements taken by the midwife this morning. 'I hope she's growing OK,' said Kate. I said reassuring things, though I have no measurements to support my belief that everything will be fine. I am part of a generation that has been taught to rely on logical reasoning rather than blind faith, on data rather than deities, but pregnancy has persuaded me that sometimes wishful thinking is better than thinking.

I was watching the evening news. Kate was watching her feet. 'I've got fat toes,' she said glumly. Today at work she had to take her socks off because they were strangling her legs.

Saturday 26 April

Kate got up and started to clean things. According to the books, this is a symptom of the nesting instinct. It hasn't affected me yet. I have the resting instinct. I went back to sleep. An hour later, she had washed everything we've been given – the pram covers, the papoose, the dog, the frog, the tortoise – and I hadn't even got out of bed.

She took her first Floradix tablet to boost her energy. I'm tempted to slip her a Valium to slow her down.

We walked to Mothercare and bought more stuff. Wet wipes. Muslin squares.

One crucial thing we haven't got yet is somewhere for our baby to sleep. We're not sure whether to use a cot or a Moses basket for the first few months. A friend came round for supper and urged us not to worry about these decisions. He spent the first months of his life in a drawer.

Kate got stuck on the sofa again. I had to haul her up.

She was itching. There are a few small itchy bumps on her skin. It is common for women to itch in the last weeks of labour, says one of the books, as the skin stretches on the abdomen. We felt reassured until we read the next paragraph. Itching can also be a symptom of obstetric cholestasis, a pregnancy-related liver disease. But this usually involves relentless itching over the entire body.

Half an hour after reading this, I was starting to itch over my entire body.

Sunday 27 April   **Week 37**

My mum phoned to say that my gran has a blood clot in the back of her brain and she still can't walk or talk normally.

My mum says that the pregnancy has brought up a lot of old, dusty memories. 'It's only since you've told me that you're having this little one. Everything that was said, it comes back to you.' She began to reminisce, filling some gaps in my knowledge of the family's history. Some of the stories were withheld from her. 'Your nana's of that generation that doesn't talk about some things. It wasn't until I was an adult that she told me I was born in a taxi.'

My mum was my gran's second child. Her first labour had been so prolonged that my gran was hoping that this birth would be quicker. To speed things along, her parents gave her castor oil. Then they went to the pub for a few hours, leaving my gran alone at home. 'When they came back from the pub,' my mum says, 'she was fully. That's why I was born in a taxi.'

When my mum was a little girl, midwives arrived on bikes. 'They went into a house with a bag. What did they have in the bag? I used to think that babies came in a bag.'

That wasn't the only misunderstanding. 'Do you remember Ray and Jean? They got married on the Saturday and the baby came on the Sunday. I thought that's what people did. I thought they got married on the Saturday and babies came on the Sunday.'

My mum doesn't remember much about my own birth. All the pain was in her back. In the end she was given a general anaesthetic and I was delivered with forceps. When she was waking up, she heard a voice saying, 'Come on, Sister, let's get this over with.' Then a doctor and a nurse showed me to my mum for the first time. She thought I had red hair. It was only later that she realised this was blood.

'He's beautiful,' said my mum.

'Come on, Mum, have a proper look,' said the doctor.

Then my mum noticed that I had a cleft lip and palate. About the staff she says, 'I can't fault them, their kindness to me.'

She was kept in Ormskirk Hospital for 18 days. It was normal practice in the mid-1960s for women to be kept in hospital for at least two weeks after the birth.

Meanwhile I was moved to a different hospital, Alder Hey. My mum couldn't sleep. One of the ward sisters told her, 'I've given you enough drugs to stop an elephant and you're still walking round all night.' Every night she paced up and down the ward. She says, 'It was like my heart had been torn out.'

I stayed in Alder Hey for six months. 'The first six months, I didn't have you. I used to go every day.' My mum was allowed to feed me except when I was recovering from surgery. After about four months the doctors repaired my cleft lip. My face was 'very very swollen'. So the nurses fed me.

For a while, after catching pneumonia, I lived in an oxygen tent.

'But you were a good baby,' said my mum, 'I couldn't fault you when you were a little one. Do you remember Mrs Blott, your teacher at St Benedict's? She said to me, "In all my years of teaching I have never met such a sweet child." And you were when you were little. I don't know what happened.' She laughed.

I was nearly killed by a dog. A poodle made of wool. As a baby I liked to suck wool, especially a poodle someone had knitted for me. Until one day my mum found a pompom in the back of my throat.

My mum's verdict on childminding: 'It's not hard work, it's just continuous.'

These are stories I've never heard before. About people I don't really know: the person I was then, and the person she was then. The pregnancy gives us another way of talking. We have something else in common. We are both parents. There are things she can begin to tell me for the first time. There are things I can better understand.

She is trying to be helpful. She asked how Kate was feeling. She said, 'Keep an eye on her ankles. Make sure her ankles don't swell up.'

I said, 'Well, I can't stop them, can I?'

'No, but it's a sign of high blood pressure. Have it checked if that happens. And watch for floaters round the eyes.'

'Floaters?'

'Little silver balls affecting your vision. That's also a sign of high blood pressure.'

Kate spent the evening in North London seeing friends. She got home at midnight and said, 'Oooh, it's nice to have a car again.'

Monday 28 April

Ian and Jacqui, whose son was born a month ago, claim that 'it is definitely worth it'. This evening I went to see for myself. They have moved to Chalfont St Giles in Buckinghamshire, half an hour from Marylebone. My train stopped at Denham Golf Club – a golf club with its own train station.

At their Parent Education classes, Ian and Jacqui were lectured by a Chinese midwife who compared the pain of childbirth to 'being stabbed in the back by a large knife'. Jacqui was terrified but the reality wasn't as bad as she feared. An epidural helped. Ian recommends gas and air, not for Kate, for me. He sneaked a few gulps when the midwife was out of the room and succumbed to giggling fits.

Since the birth, they've hardly left the house. 'Going to Tesco feels like a real achievement.' Today was Ian's first day back at work after paternity leave. He hated it. Colleagues were bringing him up to date with the office gossip and he wasn't interested. All he wanted to say was, 'Have you seen these photos of my baby?'

I held Jake while he slept. A hot little body, like he'd just come out of the oven. When he cried, his mum stuck her little finger in his mouth. He sucked fiercely until he realised that he'd been conned.

Seeing friends with their newborn baby made it seem normal and manageable. They are awed but not overawed.

I was home in bed by one o'clock in the morning. Kate said she had been worried about going into labour while she was alone.

Tuesday 29 April

We are obliged to think about life after birth. Decisions made in the first few days will affect all our lives for months or even years ahead. So we're told.

When and where should the baby sleep? None of the great ideological debates – capitalism versus communism, secular democracy versus religious autocracy – is more passionately contested than the choice between letting your baby sleep in your bed or in a cot. There are books, cited as bibles of baby care, offering conflicting commandments. Gina Ford's *The Contented Little Baby Book* provides a feeding and sleeping timetable for babies to follow. Deborah Jackson's *Three in a Bed* promotes a less strict approach and argues that sleeping with your baby is good for the whole family.

It is surprising, given that the world is full of people who know best, that the world is so fucked up. On the whole I agree with another child-rearing guru, Sheila Kitzinger, who says that 'publishers commission how-to books and say that women want clear, numbered instructions these days. They're looking for a kind of Delia Smith of child-rearing. I find that daunting – because I don't think life is like that.'

New parents are confronted by so many contradictory voices. We'll just have to do what feels right.

Even at this late stage, there is a sense of disbelief. 'I can't believe we're going to have a baby!' said Kate when she got home from work. She was cheerful and energetic. We went for a walk. I'm still waiting for her to transform into a bad-tempered ogre, a miserable housebound whale. 'People seem to think I'm huge. They keep saying, "Oh my God, you look as if you're about to pop!" The baby is kicking a lot, eager to get out. Kate has acquired a habit of rubbing her belly, like Falstaff after a satisfying meal. She does this all day. There are still anxieties. Tonight it was her nipples. 'I'm still worried that there are no holes for the milk to come out of.'

In bed I put my ear to Kate's tummy and searched. I found the baby's heartbeat, reassuringly strong and regular, low down near the belly button.

Wednesday 30 April

My stepfather was abandoned on a doorstep when he was a baby. He still has the dress he was wearing at the time. He is 6 feet 3 inches tall now. The dress is a small rag, like a napkin in his hands.

In middle age, he felt a strong urge to find his biological parents. Seeing this, my mum wondered if I would have a similar craving to find my father one day. So she gave me the address where my Italian father lived when she knew him.

A few years later, a week before my 35th birthday, I went to Italy to meet my father for the first time.

I didn't really feel a burning need to see him, just a mild curiosity. I knew that he must be in his late 50s by now. I felt that, if I was ever going to make this trip, I ought to do it soon. If I delayed for a decade or two, he might be dead by then.

I didn't let him know that I was coming. I wanted to see the look on his face when he saw me. I didn't want it to be a prepared expression. In that fraction of a second, I believed, I would get a glimpse of the real person. I wanted it to be a moment of truth. Obviously this risked hurting the people around him. It was likely that he was married with a family. He might not have told his wife and children about his English child. They might be shocked and upset. But this was a risk I was willing to take.

The address was 35 years old. It was possible that he didn't live there any more. It said Salassa, Torino. In a tourist office in Turin, Kate and I discovered that Salassa isn't a suburb of the city as we'd assumed. It is a village a train ride away.

After a night in a shabby hotel room with blue-grey walls and a stained ceiling, we boarded the morning train linking Turin to Pont Canavese. Less than an hour later, the train stopped in the middle of nowhere. This was Salassa.

It was the hottest hour of the day. We found a road, turned right and walked a mile into the village. Dogs barked at us. Even dogless houses had signs warning us to beware of the dog. As we passed a villa, with nobody else in sight, the iron gates closed automatically. Cars sped past us, heading out of town.

On Salassa's deserted main street, we saw the post office. Inside, I asked the woman behind the counter if she could direct me to the address I'd written on a piece of paper beneath my father's name: Bruno Brunasso Cassinino.

The woman examined my piece of paper and showed it to one of her colleagues and then to another customer. They all agreed that it is difficult to locate houses in this area. The house was far away on the outskirts of the village.

As she looked at the address, the woman mentioned my father's name. I heard her say to her colleague, '*Bruno è morto.*' (Bruno is dead.)

I said, '*Bruno è morto?*'

'*Sì.*'

'*Quando?*'

'*Due anni ...*' (Two years ago.)

That's how I found out my father was dead. From a woman in the post office.

Kate asked me how I felt. The truth is, we can accommodate many feelings at once. I felt frustrated that the main purpose of the journey would never be achieved. I felt disappointed that I would never meet this man. I also felt pleased that I was managing to have a conversation in Italian with real Italians.

A postman offered to take us to Bruno's old house. He drove us a couple of kilometres to the outskirts of the village where houses were scattered among the fields. We thanked the postman for his kindness and he drove off, leaving us standing outside a house next to a vineyard.

We entered the garden. It looked as if sections of the building were being renovated. We climbed the steps to a balcony with a door. I knocked. No response. A walkway extended around the side of the house. I knocked on the closed shutters. No response. A door was open. I walked into a room full of rubble and a builder's detritus. Evidently the house was empty.

We decided to explore other parts of the village. But, walking along a lane behind the house, we could hear a radio. We turned back. As we approached the grassy track leading to the gate, we noticed a middle-aged woman standing on the first-storey balcony outside her front door.

'*Buongiorno,*' I began. So far so good. I was conscious that my basic Italian lacked the nuances of language appropriate for the feelings of this situation. '*Sei la moglie di Bruno?*' (Are you Bruno's wife?)

'*Sì.*'

'*Ho sentito che Bruno è morto?*' (I've heard that Bruno died?)

'*Sì.*'

'*Mi dispiace. Bruno era un amico della mia famiglia.*' (I'm sorry. Bruno was a friend of my family.)

'*Da dove?*' (Where from?)

'*Molti anni fa, Bruno era in Inghilterra, e era un amico di mia madre.*' (Many years ago, Bruno was in England, and he was a friend of my mother's.)

As I said this, she changed. She had opened the gate to allow us into the garden. Now she took my arm and ushered us into the house. She was speaking too fast for me to understand. Kate translated.

'Yes,' said the woman, 'now I realise, I can see the resemblance.'

She couldn't have been more welcoming, more warm towards us. She led us into a dim, shuttered room on the ground floor. Her left hand was holding my right hand. We sat down. Her name was Rachele.

I asked questions in Italian. She answered in Italian. Kate translated everything I didn't understand.

I asked if she knew about me, if her husband had told her that he had an English child.

She said yes, before they married, he told her.

I could feel tears coming. I was glad the room was dark.

She said he was a good man, not 'un uomo cattivo'. (A bad man.)

I started to cry, and she cried, and Kate cried. My tears were silent but unstoppable. It was a few seconds before I could stop them. I was surprised by the emotion I felt. I still am. I don't have a word for it.

She said he had talked about me often. He had wanted to come and find me. He had bought a suitcase and said he had to go to England on his own. He told Rachele that he had loved my mother, but he had been too young. If he had been older he would have stayed.

Rachele described him fondly. He was a fit man, without a grey hair at the age of 55. He had a heart attack in the kitchen one day, and that was that, he was dead.

I thought – at least it's good news about my hair. I might die young, but at least I won't be bald.

Rachele won't go on holiday because she feels that he is still in the house and she doesn't want to abandon him. I wondered if she regarded my arrival, in a way, as a part of Bruno returning.

She spoke tenderly about him even when she was describing his faults. They met in a dance hall. Other women warned her that he wasn't the type to commit. He asked her to dance. They were together for ten years before they were married in 1974. 'He was mad,' she said, 'and I was the only one mad enough to wait for him.' Enzo, their only child, was born in 1976.

She hinted that he was a womaniser. In the final year of his life he told her that there was a 36-year-old woman who wanted to be with him. She says he refused to get involved with the 36-year-old. He was a teacher, she said, because he liked to be around young people. I guessed that meant young women in particular.

For their honeymoon, he took her for a week in the mountains. He continued to go away to mountain resorts for the holiday seasons. She said he had a different way of thinking, of seeing the world, because he had travelled a lot. He had a different mind.

A young man entered the room. He found three people with tears in their eyes. Rachele said to him, 'Do you know who this is? It is your father's son.'

He said the Italian equivalent of 'oh, right' and kissed me on each cheek. He, too, was welcoming and friendly. '*Sono contento*,' he said. (I'm pleased.) He was told about my existence two years ago, after his father's death.

We all moved upstairs into the main part of the house. Rachele gave us cake and made coffee for Kate. Kate was starving but declined an offer of food because she wasn't sure how long we ought to stay.

Rachele and Enzo showed us photos that were close at hand. Photos of Bruno and my mum in the Isle of Man. My mum looked young, glamorous in a 1960s way and happy. Then we saw photos of Rachele's wedding. Bruno's uncle had a Hitler moustache. Bruno had a uniformly serious expression in most of the photos. He was smiling only in one or two of them. Rachele wore a fluffy blue drape over her dress. It was unmistakably 1974.

Rachele gave me two photos showing Bruno in Brighton when he was 19. In one of them, he looked a bit like me.

We learnt other details about his family. Bruno's parents are both dead. Rachele and Enzo don't have much contact with Bruno's family after an argument about how to divide up a field.

Enzo said that he would like to take us to see Bruno's grave. But we talked so long that there wasn't time. We agreed to come for dinner on Monday evening, after our weekend in the mountains. We would stay the night and go to see the grave on Tuesday morning.

Back in Turin, I was thinking that I should have gone to see Bruno years ago. But I never felt the need. And what if I happened to turn up the day before his heart attack? That could have been embarrassing.

The mountains were wet and cold, so we went to visit a friend in Parma instead. On Monday, savouring the pleasures of Emilia-Romagna, we realised that we were going to be late for supper with Rachele and Enzo. We drove along the *autostrada* at recklessly illegal speeds, and we were still the slowest vehicle on the road.

At our first meeting, Rachele had said that she wasn't much of a cook. Often people say this out of false modesty. But in this case it was a simple statement of fact. She served a kind of rolled meat in an oleaginous jelly, which we felt obliged to eat. Kate, who is a food fascist, smiled and said it was nice.

Rachele showed me more photos of my father. Soon I was sick of seeing him. The more I heard about Bruno, the less I liked him. It wasn't even true, as Rachele had claimed, that he was a fit man without a grey hair on his head. He was a large man, greying and balding, with a middle-aged paunch.

Rachele gave me some presents to remember him by, although I was starting to think I'd rather forget him. She gave me one of his ties; two medals he won for playing the Italian version of boules; and a misspelt letter of reference from an Isle of Man hotel saying he was 'honest and courteous'. Bruno had framed this.

Rachele insisted on giving up her bed for us. She liked the idea of my sleeping in the bed where Bruno had slept, just as she liked me to sit at the head of the table when we ate. '*Comando come Bruno*,' she said. (In charge like Bruno.)

'*Non sono come Bruno*,' I said. (I'm not like Bruno.)

Next morning Enzo drove us all to Salto to visit Bruno's grave. Rachele mopped the floor of the burial chamber, shaped like a Swiss chalet, which Bruno shares with other members of the Cassinino family. On a plaque is a photo of Bruno aged 19, posing wistfully, looking like a prat. It wasn't the photo I would have chosen to be remembered by.

Although they had praised him loyally, Rachele and Enzo told us stories that suggested he was an egotistical and weak man.

On the eve of his father's death, Enzo gave Bruno a lift in his car. Bruno said to him, '*Guidi bene*.' (You drive well.) Enzo said this was the first compliment his father had ever paid him. Enzo was 22 years old.

With his wife, Bruno was monstrously jealous. He wouldn't allow her out of the house alone. He phoned her during the day to check what she was doing.

Early in their relationship, he took her dancing. While Bruno was talking to another woman, Rachele danced with another man. Bruno was so angry that he never took her dancing for the next 26 years. And then he died.

The next day, my 35th birthday, we went walking in the Italian Alps. Before coming to Italy, I was thinking of 35 as halfway to 70. Since finding out about Bruno's premature death, I was thinking of it as two-thirds of the way to 55.

We spent a couple of days exploring the Italian lakes. For a while I felt deflated and depressed, even tearful and angry. It was a delayed response to my encounters with Bruno's family and with Bruno himself. I considered giving back the mementos that Rachele had given me. I didn't particularly want to remember him.

We had agreed to have lunch with Rachele on our final day in Italy. I drove across northern Italy, treating the Fiat Punto like a Ferrari. In the fast lane of the *autostrada*, cars filled my rear-view mirror, indicators blinking impatiently, meaning they wanted to overtake. I was going too slowly for them. I was only doing 95mph.

During lunch, Rachele asked me if I had had a happy childhood. I had an interesting childhood, but I didn't feel like going into details. So I said, '*Avevo una madre perfetta*' and she accepted that as an answer. (I had a perfect mother.)

Rachele and her sister Donata and Enzo insisted on coming to the airport with us. They were hospitable to a fault. Taking a photograph outside the house, Kate gestured towards a tree, meaning that she wanted us to stand underneath it. Rachele misunderstood and cut off a piece of branch, thinking that Kate wanted part of the tree to take home with her.

Rachele came in the Fiat with Kate and me. Enzo and Donata followed in their own car. Rachele talked more about Bruno. I asked if he had felt guilty. She asked me to repeat the word, making sure that she had understood. '*Incolpita?*' She said he hadn't felt guilty, because he hadn't made any promises to my mum. Later, my mum told me this wasn't true.

At the airport, I went to find the place to deposit the Fiat. Enzo accompanied me. I said to him, I hope my arrival hasn't been difficult for you.

He said no, he was pleased to meet me.

I asked, with my clumsy Italian, if he was angry that his father never told him about me.

He said yes, he was a bit angry, but he felt that he would be angrier if he was in my position.

We stood awkwardly at a bar. Rachele drank orange juice that Enzo poured for her. Rachele held his coat for him.

As we said our farewells at the departure gate, Rachele spoke as if she thought I might not keep in touch. She said that I should come back again at least once. She said that Bruno would have been as pleased and proud to meet me as she was.

Rachele and Donata were crying. Donata said, 'È gli italiani.' (It's Italians.)

I wasn't crying. I said apologetically, 'Sono inglese.' (I am English.)

Next day I phoned my mum and told her that Bruno died two years ago. She tried to console me about the prospects of my own longevity. She said he was a heavy smoker. He smoked 80 a day when she knew him. I suspect she was exaggerating, but I appreciated her efforts.

I didn't tell her everything. According to Rachele, when Bruno was involved with my mother, he had an Irish girlfriend as well. Rachele thinks my mother knew about this other woman. I didn't mention it.

I said, 'His wife seems to think that he was the way he was because of his background. She says he had severe parents and he wasn't "coccolato".' This word means cuddled, cherished, loved dearly. That's why, Rachele reckons, he always felt the need to be loved.

'According to the stories I heard,' I told her, 'he was pathologically jealous.'

'Yes, he was very possessive. And everything had to be done his way.'

I said, 'Rachele asked me if I'd had a happy childhood, and I told her that I had a perfect mother.'

'Thank you.'

I said that Bruno didn't sound like one of the good guys. Whatever the difficulties she faced as a single parent, it was better than being stuck with such a weak, controlling, egocentric man. 'His wife says you had a narrow escape. And it turned out well,' I said, 'because you met Trevor, who is a hundred times the man Bruno was.'

My mum said, 'I'm going a bit weepy now.' We ended the conversation shortly afterwards.

Now I have a Christmas card relationship with Rachele and Enzo. Last December, I mentioned in the card that Kate was pregnant. Today a letter arrived from Salassa, written in formal Italian:

> Dearest Andy and Kate, for a long time we've been meaning to congrat-
> ulate you on the marvellous news that you have given. We are very happy
> about the arrival of this child and we share your joy. There are no words

to describe our emotions. With all our heart we wish so much happiness for the beautiful family you are creating. Certainly this is the most important moment in your lives, but I have no doubts about you. You have faced many struggles but the things that one obtains through effort are the most beautiful. Again, wishing so much joy to you. Sending you both a big hug, Rachele.

At the bottom of the letter is written: 'A big hug! Enzo.'

I cycled into the centre of London to meet a friend for lunch. He has just been to Paris. He asked what I've been doing. I find that I have nothing to talk about except babies and baby-related topics. I have become a baby bore. I feel like a contestant on *Mastermind* with a specialised subject but no general knowledge. I told him about the multifarious dilemmas involving car seats and prams and sleeping arrangements etc. Childless, he listened with anthropological interest. 'It's an obstacle course,' was his verdict on early parenthood.

Later I cycled between the bank, the building society and various shops, enjoying the throb and roar of the city.

You don't see many children in the centre of London. There was one today, a sulky girl in a pushchair. She threw her dummy on the floor. Her fraught mother picked it up and, eyeball to eyeball with her daughter, said, 'NOW PACK IT IN!' It wasn't the words that were threatening, it was the tone. I don't know what impact it had on the little girl, but I was scared.

Looking at the way other people are with their kids, I've decided that I want to be a calm and cheerful parent. I think this is good for the child and good for the parents. Unfortunately I'm not sure if this is something you get to choose. In his autobiography *Timebends*, Arthur Miller says that it was quite late in life that he realised how few real choices your character allows you.

Kate and I began a new era of going to Sainsbury's in the car. The parking spaces nearest the entrance are reserved for PARENT AND TODDLER PARKING. We decided that pregnant women also qualify.

Kate's brother, Phil, was staying overnight on our sofa bed. His second child will be born in July. I asked him how he's feeling about it. He said, 'It'll be a nightmare.' He expects they'll be exhausted all the time. I am gladdened by such admissions of parental misery, misgivings and mixed feelings. It's a change from the telly advert version of family life as an idyll of bonny babies and uncrumpled parents. His truthfulness makes me feel less of a misanthropic freak for having bouts of doubts. Sometimes I'm excited, sometimes I wish it wasn't happening. Every so often I think: what have I done?

I was shocked tonight when Phil asked when our baby is due and Kate replied, 'Three and a half weeks.'

I thought about it and she's right. Three and a half weeks! It sounds much nearer than 'the end of May'. Of course, it could be two weeks later than that. Or three weeks earlier.

Thursday 1 May

Months ago we were warned by friends that the Parent Education classes organised by the NHS are boring and useless, so we also booked a series of classes run by the NCT. In fact, because the midwife was enthusiastic and entertaining, we found the NHS classes enjoyable and instructive. Now we're going to see how the NCT classes compare. There are six in total, each two to four hours long, on four consecutive Thursdays and two Saturdays.

I was bored by the prospect. We've been through this stuff already. I feel like I'm ready for battle, not more training.

These classes are led by a woman called Jan. We congregated in her living room in a 1930s block of flats on Herne Hill. Five women, three men. Jan says that people make friends at these classes so that they have someone to talk to about colic and nappies and sleepless nights. 'Friends without kids,' says Jan, 'run a mile.'

Jan asked if the women have been doing their pelvic floor exercises. She said they should be doing about 50 per day. This wiped the smiles off a few faces. One woman hasn't been doing any at all. Jan said that it's the weight of the baby in the final weeks of pregnancy, not just the stress of labour, which strains the pelvic floor muscles. Pelvic floor exercises reduce the risk of long-term incontinence. 'Get squeezing,' she said. 'Walking helps, but it's not enough.' I was feeling smugly uninvolved until she said that men should do them as well to lower the chances of prostate problems in later life.

Jan made a circle out of her thumb and first finger and told us that this is the size of the uterus before pregnancy. So it expands a great deal during the nine months. The talk of labour always leads to thoughts of pain. One man shared a tip recommended to reduce the pain of labour – for the man. 'Always make sure her nails are cut short.'

Inevitably, some of Jan's information was repeating stuff we'd heard before. But there were some details that we haven't heard or have forgotten.

Jan said that pregnant women should be having regular perineal massage, with or without the help of a partner. 'Most women,' she said, 'tried it once and gave up because it was sore.' This is exactly what we did. 'You should be doing it every day for five minutes. Once a week is no good.' We did it once, three weeks ago, for two minutes. 'Remember, you are trying to create space. It's not about gently rubbing oil over the area. It's called massage because it sounds nicer. Really it should be called perineal stretch. You will find that it is quite sore at first. Try doing this and you'll get an idea.' She put a finger into each corner of her mouth and pulled. I tried this when I got home. She's right. It hurts.

Jan recommended using arnica oil or wheatgerm oil. 'You can use olive oil,' she said, 'but most people prefer something they don't use on salad. Because it puts you off salad.'

One woman thought that her baby had engaged, but she wasn't sure. She asked what it feels like. Jan said, 'You'll know when it happens. It's like walking around with a melon between your legs.' But she told us not to worry that the baby would be too big. 'Nature's way is to make babies that fit the size of the pelvis.'

We were leaping between topics. Bleeding after the birth. On average this continues for three weeks. It can go on for as long as six weeks. 'But it all sorts itself out.' This is Jan's mantra.

One woman's father has already been offering her his thoughts about names. He told her that he'll be 'very disappointed' if the baby has a traditional name. Jan said that the best thing to do with a baby's name is to keep it to yourself until it is born. Once it is on the birth certificate, family and friends are less likely to offer unhelpful opinions.

Jan recommends that pregnant women should take Floradix from 36 weeks onwards. She also says that men should take it as well, to boost our iron and energy levels for the exhausting weeks ahead of us.

One myth that Jan was keen to dispel is that first babies usually come late. She said that it's about half and half. 'Half come before the due date, half come after.'

This made Kate worried. As we walked to the car, she said, 'If I'd known that, I would've stopped work earlier.' Our pregnancy is more advanced than any of the others, but all the other women have stopped work already.

This wasn't her only anxiety. She had been comparing bumps. She said to me, 'I feel like I've got the smallest belly.'

I tried to be reassuring. 'You haven't. They're just fat.' I felt like I was being unfairly cruel to my new friends.

Tonight we went to see a recording of *Have I Got News For You?* with a group of old friends. One of them said to Kate, 'You're looking very big.'

'That's nice to hear,' she said.

Friday 2 May

Met friends for lunch. A noisy Thai restaurant on Wardour Street.

Rob has placed an advertisement on several dating websites. He is pretending to be a woman called Alice. Alice describes herself as mid-20s, blonde and single. Alice says that, as a personal assistant to a businessman, she travels all over the world. Alice says that, following the break-up of a long relationship, she is looking for a more casual relationship with the right kind of man. Alice says that the man she wants doesn't have to be amazingly handsome or rich. What appeals to Alice, what turns her on, is a man who is good with words. The last line of her advertisement is: 'Write to me and seduce me.'

Rob/Alice is receiving 10–20 emails per day. Some men write romantic poems. Some messages are extremely pornographic. The American men are more sexually suggestive than the British men. Some of the men mention that they are married. Rob says that this enterprise has convinced him that men are twats. He is going to compile the best replies in a book called *Seducing Alice*.

I almost said to him, 'But you can't call this slag Alice, that's my daughter's name.'

At home Kate lay on the sofa, swollen ankles raised on pillows. In bed, we tried an experiment. I listened to the regular thumping of the baby's heartbeat. I wondered if it's possible to tape it so that Kate can hear it as well. So I placed a Dictaphone against the bump and pressed 'Record'. When we played it back we could hear a regular tapping noise with the fast rhythm of our baby's heartbeat. We played it back several times, savouring the sound of our baby. Then we got suspicious and recorded the silent room. When we played that back, the regular tapping noise was still there. It wasn't a heartbeat at all. It was just the clicking of the Dictaphone's own mechanism.

Kate was tearful before sleep. She said that she didn't know why. She didn't sleep well. Aching hips. Pains in her lower back. Turning over is an effort.

Saturday 3 May

We missed our second NCT class to go to a wedding. Kate has borrowed a maternity dress from a friend. She scowled at herself in the mirror. 'I'm fat!'

'You're not fat, you're pregnant.'

She dropped her mobile phone. She tripped over the door wedge. At last we were sitting in the car. I turned the key in the ignition and Kate said, 'We haven't locked the door.' I looked and saw that the front door of the house was wide open. We're too stupid to be parents.

It was an unorthodox wedding in many ways. The happy couple arrived together and mingled with the guests for an hour before the ceremony. They had written their own vows and chosen their own music; the ceremony began with Handel and ended with Elvis. There was a best man and a best woman. Seventy guests sat on one side of the church on three rows of chairs, facing another seventy guests on three rows of chairs on the other side of the church. In the aisle between the guests, the happy couple and their dog sat facing the vicar. Afterwards, everyone strolled around Battersea Park for an hour while photographs were taken. Then we returned to the church for a meal. Some guests cooked the food; other guests did the washing-up.

The bride looked elegant. So did the other bride. Clare wore a pink-patterned silk blouse and Nina wore a three-quarter-length cream coat. Despite personal reservations, one bride's mother attended the ceremony and the other bride's mother turned up during the food and speeches. Some family members didn't attend because they disapproved of two women marrying each other, but their absence didn't spoil the day. All weddings are an embodiment of love. This wedding was also an embodiment of courage, challenging a society that tries to impose limits on who and how we love.

Kate was public property all day. In between songs, the wedding singer put her head against the bump and tried to listen to the baby. Kate was closely observed by a wedding guest who has been cast as a pregnant woman in a play and who wanted to analyse how she walked. Strangers touched her belly; friends discussed her swollen toes.

As the wedding photographer, I didn't have much time to chat to people. When I did, I found the men talking less about football and more about babies than they used to. Greg – a father of a little girl – assured me that birth is a fantastic experience, though he admitted that his wife didn't enjoy it as much as he did. She didn't shout much; she just held his hand and crushed it. He already had an idea of what to expect because his own mother had described childbirth to him. His mother said, 'Take your top lip and pull it over the top of your head. That's how painful it is.'

Kate's body continues to be a source of amazement to her and me. In bed, lying on her back, she said, 'Look at my tits!' Her nipples were pointing at the ceiling instead of the walls. 'It's like I've had implants.'

She stared at her belly. 'She's been very quiet. I don't know whether to be worried. She hasn't moved very much.'

Sunday 4 May   Week 38

Another disturbed night for Kate. Heartburn. Sore hips. She thinks the baby has moved lower. We tried to feel the baby's head. We found it, a hardness under the skin, but then we found similar hardnesses in different places. Our baby has three heads. The truth is, we can't tell her arse from her elbow.

'She's moving loads!' said Kate happily.

A group of friends from yesterday's wedding, including the two brides, met for lunch at Café Rouge in Clapham. The childless people arrived on time. The pregnant people were 15 minutes late. The people with children were half an hour late.

Someone asked us, 'Have you packed your bag yet?' People have been asking us this all weekend. It's one of the standard questions asked of pregnant people, but it's making us anxious because we haven't packed the bag yet.

We should pack the bag. It is the first day of week 38 already. If our baby were born now she wouldn't be regarded as premature. She could arrive at any time in the next five weeks. Birth, like death, sneaks up on you.

One friend, a mother of two, advises us to arrange a social event for the evening that our baby is due to be born. She suggests booking a meal in a restaurant. Something that will reduce expectation and disappointment if the baby fails to appear on that day.

After lunch (steak and champagne) we walked to Clapham Common. Kate escorted the toddlers into the busy playground and emerged with post-traumatic stress disorder. A mother warned us, 'Waiting for children to leave the playground is the most boring thing in the world.' A father agreed: 'It's fun at first, then the novelty wears off. "Push me! Push me! Push me!"'

Cleo, aged three, said, 'It's so windy my nose is going to blow off.' It was windy enough to fly kites. Kate exposed her belly to the sun and the women gathered round to touch it.

'You're big now!' said Sophie. Kate is happy to hear this. It corroborates the pregnancy. But using the right vocabulary is important. She wasn't so gratified today when Nina said, 'You *are* fat!'

The wedding day has become a wedding weekend. We had supper at the brides' house and watched them opening their presents. This must be how Muslims feel at Christmas.

I enjoyed today. But back home, Kate complained tearfully that I'd been looking grumpy-faced all day. She wants me to be more 'relaxed'. And it's true that in general I am feeling tense and worried, mostly because of frustrations related to my job and my financial prospects and my ability to fulfil my parental responsibilities. I'm trying not to be too miserable but I can't spend my days pretending to be what I'm not. Women complain that men don't communicate their feelings enough. And then they complain when we look pissed off.

Monday 5 May

When we woke up, Kate apologised for berating me last night. 'I'm sorry for being upset. I'm just emotional.'

A bank holiday. I made a list. Sainsbury's, IKEA, towel rail, pram, light switch, windows, bathroom floor, shelving, chest of drawers …

I'm emotional too. I was in a bad mood because I wanted to do some work at my desk but I had to put up the towel rail.

'Don't do it if you don't want to,' said Kate.

'When will it get done, then? This is life from now on. Doing things you don't want to do.'

I remember thinking months ago that my role is to make Kate as happy as possible while she's pregnant. I'm not doing very well. She was in tears again. She said that she was worried about how much we're arguing, and worried that we'll argue when the baby is here.

I apologised for my grouchiness. I screwed the towel rail to the wall and went to Sainsbury's. By then, most of the afternoon had gone. In bleaker moments, I imagine the rest of life being like this, an endless succession of chores leaving us no time to be loving or lovable. Having children is either the best thing I've ever done or the worst mistake of my life. I'm still not sure which.

Her friend Iris phoned. She has given birth to a girl. This came as a surprise to Iris because she was told after the second scan that it was a boy.

Kate is being tortured by her own body. Today she felt a burning in her vagina around the perineum, like a stretching. Tonight she grimaced with heartburn. She felt as if she had swallowed a hot poker.

I had just gone to bed with a book when she said, 'I might just do a perineal massage.'

'With or without my help?' I tried to seem sincere and arranged my face in something resembling a warm smile.

'You don't seem enthralled by the prospect.'

'I'm sure neither one of us is enthralled by it.'

'I'll just do it myself.'

Tuesday 6 May

My producers sent the script to the actor Ralph Fiennes, via his agent, nearly two months ago. If Ralph Fiennes says that he wants to play the lead role, the movie will get made. I was told that Mr Fiennes had read the script and liked it. But he wanted to see a video of the director's work before agreeing to a meeting. Videos were sent to him. We waited. And waited. After seven weeks of waiting, I heard today that 'Ralph Fiennes has passed'. 'Passed' is a euphemism for 'said no'. No explanation was given. Two months wasted. Now they're going to approach Kenneth Branagh. More waiting.

I told Kate the bad news when she got home from work. About ten minutes later she gave me a hug and said that she loved me. Maybe she was trying to cheer me up. It worked.

Played football in Brixton. Among the fathers, opinions differ about what the impact will be on my football career. Rod, father of two, said, 'We won't be seeing much of you, then.' Bobby, father of one, said, 'I didn't miss a week.'

Kate said that the baby wasn't moving much. She wanted me to listen to its heartbeat. I found it in the usual place, 2 inches south-east of her belly button.

She said, 'Can you hear it?'

'Yeah.'

'How does it sound?'

'Completely normal.' I tapped her bottom to imitate the fast rhythm of the baby's heart. Taptaptaptaptaptaptaptaptaptaptaptap.

She looked relieved. 'I've been having a strange feeling.'

'What kind of feeling?'

'Up to now I've felt that she's better off inside me, but now's the first time I feel that she's better off outside me.' I nodded as if I understood. 'I don't want to damage her by keeping her in there.'

'You're not damaging her, lovey, you're feeding her and helping her to grow.'

'I didn't say it was rational.'

Wednesday 7 May

I've decided to go to Warrington to visit my gran in the hospital. Kate was keen for me to travel sooner rather than later, in case the baby comes early.

I like sitting on trains and writing, but these days it's almost impossible because of the number of people talking on mobile phones. I was surrounded by four business people. They seemed to be competing with each other. When one of them made a phone call, the others needed to feel important and started phoning people as well. One woman hadn't acquired the knack of moderating her voice. SHE WAS SHOUTING ALL THE TIME. I wouldn't have minded if her conversation was interesting. I heard her giving her phone number to a work colleague. I made a note of it and sent her a text message from my own phone. I wrote: 'Please don't shout on the phone.'

Nana looked dead when I saw her. She was lying flat on the bed, corpse-like. Her body was pale and blue-veined, swollen and shrivelled. Her older brother, Uncle Edmund, was sitting at her bedside. I asked him how he was. He said he was fine. I knew this wasn't true. He has been ill. His wife, Aunty Lil, has also been unwell.

I listened to Uncle Edmund and Nana talking about their friends.

'How's Martha?' asked Uncle Edmund.

'She's not a good colour.'

'How's Elizabeth?'

'Not so good.'

'I heard she wasn't well.'

'I don't think any of them are, do you?' said Nana.

Her speech was slurred, difficult to understand. The blood clot is in one of the small arteries in her brain, affecting balance, speech and swallowing. For two weeks she has been recuperating in a hospital room on her own. This morning the staff moved her to a ward with seven other elderly women to encourage her to interact more. The other patients can't understand what she says. She said to me, 'I miss our conversations.' We used to sit in her flat and discuss the world. Today we sat mostly in silence. 'I'm not much company,' she said. She became tired quickly so I left her alone to doze for an hour. In the canteen I ate a pie, chips and beans, good Northern food. When I returned to the ward, Nana was eating lamb casserole. She didn't want it, but she finished it. I had to open her banana for her. She was too weak.

I watched women being craned out of bed, lifted out of chairs by heavy machinery, strapped to trolleys and wheeled to the toilet. Each withered body was crowned by an immaculate hairdo. A hairdresser tours the ward every day.

When the nurses were out of the room, the old ladies grumbled. One of them was waiting for her colostomy bag to be changed. A woman called Mary told her, 'They don't come unless you ask.'

'I don't like to ask.'

'I know, you get frightened, don't you?'

Nana wanted her slippers on. I struggled to squeeze them over her swollen feet. She sat in a chair at the side of her bed and smiled at other patients. But it wasn't her usual smile – it was a disconcerting grin, as if she had ingested a happy drug. I chose a coherent moment to give her a photo of Kate and the bump and me, and she seemed pleased. She told me to put it in her handbag where it would be safe. She said, 'Maybe next time I see you, you'll have your baby.' I was glad that she believes there will be a next time. She isn't giving up.

Aunts, uncles and cousins came to visit. It was my uncle's 42nd wedding anniversary recently. He says, 'Even the Krays only got 35 years.'

Among the men, the talk was of pubs and the price of beer. My cousin said that he is going to join 'the cons club'.

'What's that?' I asked.

'The Conservative Club,' he said.

My uncle, who is already a member, elaborated. 'When it's happy hour, you get a pint for 75 pence.'

I suspect that my uncles would join the Nazi Club if it had cheap beer.

I showed them the photos of Kate and the bump. They all said it looked like twins and laughed.

Train, tube, bus. Back in Peckham before midnight. An email from New Zealand. Kate's friend Wendy has given birth to a little boy. It was a traumatic experience. The baby's eye was damaged during a forceps delivery.

They don't know if the cornea will heal or not. Wendy needed a blood transfusion. That was eight weeks ago. She says she has only just recovered. She tells us, 'Be prepared for more arguments.'

Thursday 8 May
One couple failed to attend this morning's NCT class. The woman is only 35 weeks pregnant but was admitted to hospital last week because her waters broke. She wasn't having contractions so she was sent home again. Her baby currently weighs about 5½ pounds, so it has a good chance of survival even if it is born this early. Our teacher, Jan, tells us that another couple, also 35 weeks pregnant, went to Paris for the weekend. The woman went into labour and gave birth in a hospital there. These stories widened everyone's eyes.

Jan gave us a list of things to take into hospital. It was similar to the list we've compiled, with a couple of interesting additions. *Pillows.* You'd think that a hospital would have pillows, but apparently there's a shortage because patients take them home. *A bendy straw.* Picking up a cup suddenly seems like a lot of trouble. *Bath and toilet seat cleaner.* 'I really wouldn't sit on the loos in hospital without wiping them over with antiseptic wipes.'

Today's class was about pain management. Jan said that in all her years of teaching, only two women have said that childbirth didn't hurt at all.

There were groans of disbelief and envy. Everyone in the class hated those two women.

Unlike every other pain in life, said Jan, 'this is a positive pain, a useful pain, each contraction is one less, bringing you closer to your baby. Don't forget it's about the baby, don't forget the end result. Otherwise you can get worn down. Don't be a martyr. If you do need some pain relief, take it.'

We discussed the different options, stuff we'd heard before.

Hiring a birthing pool to use at home costs about £200. One woman gave birth in a Deluxe Paddling Pool from John Lewis because it was cheaper.

Some women say that a birthing pool gave them 'incredible pain relief', but this fails to sway one woman in our group who says she can't use a birthing pool because she hates her fingers going wrinkly in water.

Gas and air. 'A lot of people say it just wasn't enough.' 'The more relaxed you are, the more effective things are.' 'The main thing is positive thinking.'

Pethidene. 'It can make you sleepy. It makes some women feel scared. It might be a really good trip or a really bad trip. Some babies are injected with an antidote because they come out so floppy. The effects of pethidene on the baby can be noticeable for seven days after the birth.' Another drawback to pethidene is that some mothers are too dopey to appreciate the moment of birth. They can be emotionally numbed and indifferent when meeting their baby for the first time.

Epidurals. These days a low dosage epidural is given for women in labour. This means you can still feel your legs. The dosage is timed, ideally, to wear off by the second stage of labour so that you're able to push. But an epidural also means that you'll be attached to a drip to stabilise your blood pressure, a catheter inserted vaginally and a belt monitor for continual assessment of the baby's condition.

I asked Jan which she would recommend, if it came to a choice between pethidene and an epidural.

'An epidural,' she said. 'At least then, mentally, you're with it.'

We talked about birth plans. This is a wish list, a description of the type of birth you'd like to have. It's like a letter to Santa Claus. You might be lucky, you might get what you want. If nothing else, a birth plan gives guidance to the maternity staff and lets them know that you have an informed opinion about the birth process. According to Jan, 'Midwives say the majority of people they see don't have a clue about anything. They haven't been to classes. They haven't read the books. The problem then is that midwives are more likely to take decisions without consulting you. You get railroaded through the system.'

But we mustn't be too rigid in our expectations. Jan told a disturbing story about a woman who told her partner that she didn't want any pain relief under any circumstances, even if she was screaming for it. Sure enough, the labour was protracted and the woman asked for an epidural. Her partner overrode the request and kept waving the piece of paper she'd signed renouncing pain relief. The midwives were reluctant to intercede because of the risk of being sued. Eventually the baby became distressed and the doctors intervened and performed an emergency Caesarean. Three months later, the parents split up.

A birth plan doesn't give us control of the process, but it gives us an influence. That's the theory. I told a friend who works in the NHS that we were preparing a birth plan and he laughed. 'Yes, they have to have something to ignore.'

The other people in the class asked occasional questions and made infrequent contributions. I passed on a tip I'd read somewhere. A tennis ball makes a good back massager. People wrote it down. 'Tennis ball.' I felt good. This is my small contribution to alleviate suffering in the world. Jan said, put the tennis ball in a sock if it feels scratchy on your skin.

'I'm starting to get bored,' said Kate after the class. Most of this stuff we've heard before.

I drove Kate to the Institute of Psychiatry where she was sitting a Family Therapy exam this afternoon. She said later that, in the middle of the exam, she felt wetness between her legs and was scared that her waters were breaking. She thought, 'Not now, Alice, not now.' It turned out to be nothing, a false alarm, a fantasy, a moment of exam hysteria.

I read in the catalogue that Mothercare shops hire out TENS machines, so I went along to the Peckham branch. I said to an assistant there, 'Excuse me, I'm looking for information about hiring TENS machines.'

She turned to her colleagues for help. 'TENS machines?'

Four women looked at me. 'What do you want?'

'I want to hire a TENS machine,' I said.

'Oh yeah,' said one of the women, remembering. 'It's a breast pump, innit?'

'Er, no, it's for pain relief.'

'Sorry,' said another woman, 'we don't do it any more.'

In Boots they were more knowledgeable. The woman there said that I could hire a machine called a BABY TENS. Unfortunately she didn't have any in stock, and didn't know when more would be available.

It was all a waste of time anyway. Kate phoned the NCT and hired a TENS machine from them. It costs £28 for a month plus £4 for delivery. It arrives on Monday morning.

Kate's piano teacher, Sam, says that she and her husband, who is also called Sam, induced the birth of their child by having sex three weeks after the due date. But she says it was an unpleasant experience for both of them. 'We felt like animals.'

Kate thinks that Alice has changed sides. There is aching in her lower back, more pressure on her bladder.

Friday 9 May

Kate has given up going to the cinema. She can't sit still for that long.

It could be worse. A pregnant friend feels nauseous when she swallows her own saliva. She is spitting her way through pregnancy. At home, she spits. In the street, she spits. In restaurants, she spits. Because spitting is better than vomiting.

We drove to the hospital for the first time, trying to find a route with a minimum number of speed bumps. Kate glowers at me when the car goes over one. Today I found a solution. I let her drive.

We sat in the waiting room with a scattering of other pregnant women. Like a scene from *Invasion of the Body Snatchers*. Kate has a habit of going for a glass of water from the cooler and bringing one for me, depriving me of an opportunity to be useful, and making me look like a lazy twat. Today she was too heavy to move, so I heroically went to fetch the water. Our appointment was at nine o'clock. At 10.50, Kate's name was called.

The midwife said, 'My name's Mildred.'

'We saw you two weeks ago,' said Kate.

'You probably remember me because I talk a lot,' said Mildred. 'How are you feeling?'

Kate mentioned that she has had pains in her knees and hips, especially at night.

That's because of the weight of the baby, said Mildred, and hormones are softening the ligaments in preparation for labour.

'Is there anything I can do?' asked Kate.

'You can have a hot bath before bed,' said Mildred. 'But you'll still get the pains. You can't win.'

We asked her to show us where to put the pads for the TENS machine on Kate's back. She showed me two places on Kate's lower back, either side of the sacrum where the nerves emerge from the bone, and a couple of places higher up. She let me feel the sacrum. Then she showed me one last time. Either side of the sacrum. 'And here.' She put her fingers in a completely different place from the previous time.

Kate said she thinks the baby has changed position.

At first Mildred disagreed. Then she felt around. 'Oh you're right you know.' She declared that the baby isn't lying on the left or the right any more. She is lying in the middle, on her back, with her spine against Kate's spine. 'That's why you're getting a lot of backache. She's lying back to back. She's probably praying. She's like this.' For half a second Mildred did an impression of our baby lying on her back, arms flailing above her. 'But that doesn't mean she's going to stay there.'

We listened to the heartbeat. One hundred and fifty beats per minute.

Mildred sat down and filled in the antenatal report. She asked if we've been to any classes.

'Yes,' said Kate.

'OK, what do you do if you feel wetness between your legs?'

I searched my brain for the answer. It was full of buckets and tennis balls. I knew what TENS stood for. Transcutaneous Electrical Nerve Stimulation. But I couldn't actually recall anything of practical benefit. Luckily I wasn't the one on the spot.

There was a silence. Kate said, 'Go to the hospital.'

'No,' said Mildred. 'You go to the toilet and pee. If you can stop the flow, it's just urine. If you can't stop the flow, it's your waters. It smells different.'

I said, 'We were told that it's very rare for the waters to break before you're 8 centimetres dilated.'

'No,' said Mildred, 'your waters can break anytime from week 24, or they might not break until just before the baby comes out.' This wasn't what the other midwife had said. I'm sure it wasn't. By now the problem is that we've read so much and heard so much that every piece of information contradicts something else we've been told. We are looking for certainty and predictability, yet it seems that even giving birth is a matter of opinion.

Mildred didn't seem impressed by the quality of our learning. We departed feeling like naughty schoolchildren who had failed an elementary test.

Our priorities are all wrong. We still haven't packed the bag for the hospital. We still haven't written a birth plan. But we have bought picture frames.

Kate had the same thought. At home she said, 'What if I go into labour tonight? We haven't got a bag packed or anything!'

It's true that she could go into labour tonight, but I'm having trouble really believing it. Despite all the books and classes and equipment, the baby is still an abstract concept.

My lack of belief doesn't alter the fact that it's true. This time tomorrow we could be living with a baby.

Kate massaged and stretched her perineum for five minutes. She said, 'God, it's a bit frightening! The pain! Even just stretching it is painful.'

Pain and fear are coming up in conversation more often. Kate is seeking help wherever she can get it. She examined the homeopathy pills that a friend gave us to use during labour and the hours beforehand. There's a pill called Aconite 200. The leaflet claims that it 'Reduces fear, anxiety and panic. Can be taken before labour if fearful about the event.'

I said, 'You're not panicking, are you? You don't need it.'

'I do need it.'

'What is it?'

'I don't know. But whatever it is, I need it.'

Saturday 10 May

I know from riding a motorbike and having sex (not at the same time) that instruction manuals just can't convey what the activity really feels like, and I strongly suspect that parenthood belongs to that same category of incommunicable experience. No book or video or class can convey the reality of having a baby. I'm tired of this phoney war. I'm ready for battle. I'm bored by the baby books, the bornography. I want the real thing now.

The flat is a mess. Full of clutter. Carrycots, car seats, mattresses, pillows, bouncing chairs, baby carriers with straps, unassembled furniture in boxes. We look like we've just moved in. I suppose that's what we're doing. Moving into our new life.

We went into central London to buy more things. Towels. A bathrobe for Kate.

In the evening, a friend phoned and we arranged to meet in a pub in Camden. His girlfriend is starting to talk about having kids. He doesn't feel ready and doesn't know if he ever will. He has male friends who say they do feel certain about their desire to have a family and this makes him wonder if his own uncertainty is a temporary state of mind or a permanent aspect of his temperament.

If he was looking for an answer, he was asking the wrong person. Luckily he knows me well enough not to expect wisdom. Instead I referred him to Thomas Hardy who mocked the notion of permanence when he described the marriage of Jude the Obscure: 'And so, standing before the [parson], the two swore that at every other time of their lives till death took them, they would assuredly believe, feel, and desire precisely as they had believed, felt, and desired during the few preceding weeks. What was as remarkable as the undertaking itself was the fact that nobody seemed at all surprised at what they swore.'

I don't think I made my friend feel better; if anything, I made things worse. I suggested that, although I can't be certain about this, a degree of ambivalence is a natural state of mind for most people. If you're lucky, you can choose the kind of life you live. Having made the choice, you can't help wondering now and again how you'd be getting along in those alternative lives that you didn't choose. It isn't the actual alternatives that you crave, it's the feeling of having choices available, the feeling that life stretches ahead with a broad horizon of possibilities. When you lose this, you're left with a sense of lostalgia. It takes time getting used to that.

Don't count your blessings. Just enjoy them. That's the secret. Otherwise, you end up like Baudelaire. He said: *'Je suis toujours bien là où je ne suis pas.'* (I am always happy wherever I am not. Happiness is always somewhere else.)

Sunday 11 May   **Week 39**

While I was at the pub last night, Kate was packing The Bag. There are so many things that we're supposed to take to the hospital. The Bag is actually three bags. Stuff for the baby. Stuff for Kate. Stuff for me.

I typed out the birth plan on the computer and printed it. It looks beautiful, a white page patterned with neat black type. Sections have been underlined, indented and justified. The headings are in bold. Our birth plan is clean and tidy, nicely structured and not too long. Everything that birth isn't, I'm sure.

'What's a birth plan?' asked Drew, who came round for lunch. Somehow he has become a father of two children without ever writing a birth plan.

His first child arrived after a 24-hour labour. 'I was just an emotional punchbag,' he told me. 'I was either holding her hand or being told to fuck off.'

He wished us well for the birth and assured us that parenthood will be 'interesting'.

'Interesting?'

'Well …' We waited for him to elaborate. He possibly felt under pressure to provide words of comfort or inspiration. 'We're no wiser than anybody else.' The words, on the tip of his tongue, toppled off the edge. 'It's one of the most fantastic times as well as one of the most difficult.'

Drew almost missed the birth. He was working in Madrid until a day before his son was born. This reminded me that, whatever the financial perils of self-employment, at least I can make sure I'm around.

But there are some advantages to being a wage slave. Wages, for example. And also Drew said: 'It was nice going on the occasional business trip because it meant I could get a night's sleep.'

Monday 12 May

This evening we read the instructions for the TENS machine. You're supposed to test it as soon as you get it, so I placed the four electrode pads on Kate's back and attached the wires to a compact control box smaller than a Walkman. It felt like a peculiarly electronic procedure, as if we were assembling a hi-fi rather than having a baby. When it was time to switch on the machine, Kate said warily, 'Can I do the next bit?' She turned the dials tentatively. She was meant to feel a pinprick sensation on her back.

'Can you feel it?'

'Are you touching me?' she accused.

'No.'

'I can feel it, then. It's more like a finger stroke than a pinprick.'

She experimented with the controls. She said it felt like a series of small electric shocks. They can be intermittent or continuous, and there's a booster button for when the pain gets really excruciating. A TENS machine is supposed to encourage the production of the body's natural painkillers. Judging by Kate's expression, she wasn't entirely convinced. She finds it bizarre, the concept of giving herself electric shocks.

After a couple of minutes she turned off the power and I unpeeled the electrode pads. We're not sure they were in the right place on her back. She said she felt queasy and her legs were trembling. We don't know if this was a side effect of the electric shocks or just the thought of what's to come.

She was still frowning at the machine. I reminded her what the midwife said: 'The more you relax, the more effective things are.' Easy for me to say.

When I went into the bedroom, she still looked troubled. She was lying on her back, legs apart, gingerly stretching her perineum.

She said, 'How's a baby ever going to come out of that? Look at that hole.' I looked at the hole. She kindly pulled it to its maximum diameter, about 1½ inches across. I imagined the size of the baby's head. I can see why she finds it so hard to feel relaxed about the whole process.

Tuesday 13 May
Delivered a script and two story ideas to the BBC offices near Oxford Circus. Spent the afternoon wallowing in central London. I invited Louise along. She agreed to come, she said, 'because it's probably the last time' that I'll be available for any social activity for the foreseeable future. Louise said that labour is like a roller-coaster ride, and once you're on it you can't get off.

We went to the V&A where I asked a member of staff for directions to the exhibition of 20th-Century Propaganda Posters.

He said, 'Do you know where the Frank Lloyd Wright Room is?'

'No.'

'It's above there.'

I came home from Oxford Street with a wooden rocking frame to support the carrycot, a mini-deckchair to support the baby in the bath, a bath thermometer in the shape of a fish and sunshades for the car windows.

Kate has noticed wistfully that her legs are losing their shape as they swell. They look like table legs. Two thick stumps with fat toes.

She reported happily that the baby has 'been kicking loads all day'. A friend at work, who hadn't seen her for a few days, remarked that the bump is definitely lower than it was a week ago.

Any day now.

Every so often, in the middle of a conversation about breast pumps or nappy liners, a thought comes into my head. 'I should be hiking in Peru.' 'I haven't seen the Great Barrier Reef.' But on reflection – maybe I'm fooling myself – I can't think of a bigger adventure than having a baby.

Wednesday 14 May
Getting dressed is posing new challenges for Kate. Her feet can only fit into sandals now. She only has two pairs of socks that don't dig into her ankles.

Bran Flakes on the kitchen table. She is constipated again.

This afternoon she attended a breastfeeding workshop for four hours. It was conducted by an entertaining Irish woman in her 60s, Sinead, who said that her first exposure to breastfeeding was as a child in Ireland when she saw a tinker woman clasping a baby to her chest. The word 'chest' was preferred in those days. The word 'breast' was never heard. Sinead's mother, shocked, told her off for even looking at those 'dirty people'.

Statistics suggest that breastfeeding isn't as easy as it looks. After the birth of their baby, 69 per cent of mothers breastfeed. Within a week, the figure has fallen to 55 per cent. After 2 weeks, it's 52 per cent. After 6 weeks, it's 42 per cent. After 4 months, it's 28 per cent. After 6 months, it's 21 per cent.

Most mothers say they wished they could have breastfed for longer. Reasons for giving up in the first 6 weeks/6 months include 'insufficient milk' (39 per cent/44 per cent), pain (25 per cent/6 per cent), the baby wouldn't suck/rejected the breast (24 per cent/11 per cent), it took too long (18 per cent/14 per cent), illness in mother or baby (16 per cent/8 per cent), returned to work (1 per cent/26 per cent), other reasons (14 per cent/22 per cent).

Antenatal yoga was strenuous tonight. Kate says she had to abandon some of the positions earlier than the other women.

Each day is filled with chores and obligations. There's always more to be done, always this feeling that I'm behind.

Thursday 15 May
An electrician came round last week. He has sent us a quote for installing a light in the bathroom (there is already a live wire there) and fitting a pull cord. He wants £178 plus VAT. He can fuck off.

We thought about missing this morning's four-hour NCT class. Kate has lots of things to finish at work and so do I. But in the end we went along. And it was worth it. You pick up little details that make you feel more prepared for what might happen.

According to Jan, induction is a procedure that's open to negotiation. Jan says it's not inevitable that you'll need to be induced after 42 weeks. 'I know a woman who went to 44 weeks.'

I've heard different rules from different midwives about when the waters break. Jan's opinion is: 'There's no rule.' Sometimes midwives break the waters with a hook. Jan says they often don't have a medical reason for this; they're just trying to speed up the birth and we don't have to accept that. 'If they break your waters, your contractions become much more uncomfortable.'

Jan thinks it's best to let things take their natural course. 'Induction is likely to lead to further interventions. Induction is the beginning of the cascade of intervention. It's a slippery slope.'

There are alternative methods to initiate the labour. She mentions caloferum, clary sage, acupuncture, spicy food, castor oil ('as a last resort, it tastes horrible') and sex.

Nipple stimulation can also be effective, but she warns that 'It's not one quick tweak, it's a long process, about an hour at a time.'

'An hour!' exclaimed Kate.

Jan continued. 'It's important to do one nipple at a time. Doing both nipples at the same time can distress the baby.' Sometimes I think she's making things up.

A late labour poses tormenting dilemmas. 'You have to hope that you get a midwife who offers positive input.' Jan said that, after years of experience of hundreds of births, she has found that 'Women who don't progress straight away don't progress later on.' But it's difficult to abandon hope of a natural labour. 'It's like waiting for a bus. You think, you've waited this long, it must be just around the corner.'

Jan talked about the use of forceps and ventouse. 'With a forceps delivery, it's common for doctors to put a foot on the bed and pull forcefully.' Someone gasped. 'I'm telling you so that, if it happens, you know what might be involved. For the woman, the hormones take over. Sometimes it's more disturbing for the birthing partner who can see what's going on. It's a frightening thing to witness.'

If we end up having an emergency Caesarean, 'it isn't like an episode of ER'. Doctors and nurses running dramatically down corridors, stethoscopes flying, only happens in 1 per cent of cases. Dad is allowed to be present at a Caesarean unless a general anaesthetic is being used. He'll be given a gown and a hat to wear, the uniform of the operating theatre. To avoid being mistaken for a member of staff and offered a scalpel, he'll be given a label saying DAD. There is a 'nice, positive atmosphere' and the operation takes about 10 minutes or less, leaving a 10-centimetre scar above the bikini line. There is music playing; if you don't like the doctor's choice, you can request a change, Jan says. Personally, even if they were playing heavy metal, I don't think I'd notice.

After a Caesarean, the mother is kept in for two to three days in an NHS hospital, or five days in a private hospital. Dads aren't supposed to spend the night on the post-natal ward. 'That would be the official line,' says Jan, 'but just say no and wait for them to get security. If you have a sensible midwife, she'll let the father stay. She'll just pull the curtain around the bed and pretend he isn't there.'

After a break for sandwiches and bananas and peeing, we moved on to the next subject. Breastfeeding. Jan says that one of the benefits for the mother 'is a sense of pride that you've grown this little person'.

Jan debunked some breastfeeding myths. Breastfeeding isn't a reliable contraceptive. Some people think it is, and find themselves back on the labour ward within a year of the first birth.

All breasts are capable of producing enough milk to feed a baby. Size doesn't matter. Abigail protested sorrowfully, 'Why have I got huge breasts, then? Why have I had to acquire these monsters? They've trebled in size. They used to be quite modest.' Jan could offer no consolation. Even Abigail's breasts have the same number of milk ducts as everyone else's.

In the early days, a baby will probably need feeding about every three hours. Sometimes you have to wake it up by tickling its feet. Jan shares my opinion that the approach of people like Gina Ford, the author of *The Contented Little Baby Book*, who urge parents to impose a strict feeding and sleeping timetable on babies, is too militaristic. 'Gina Ford is a Nazi,' said Jan. 'Gina Ford hasn't got children of her own. It's easier to leave children crying when they're not your own. If it's your child, it's like having a knife stuck in you.'

Mothers who breastfeed require an extra 500 calories per day. It's the partner's job to keep the fridge stocked with grabbable, instantly eatable food. Heating something in a pan will seem like too much trouble. Jan says she used to carry a tuck box full of sandwiches and biscuits. One of the disadvantages of breastfeeding, her husband found, is crumbs in the bed.

We were given cards containing statements about breastfeeding. We had to say whether they were true or false. One podgy man read out, 'Breastfeeding will ruin your figure.' He paused. 'Well, I don't think it'll ruin mine. I've already done that myself.'

It took me almost three hours to replace the broken dimmer switch in the bedroom and to install a light in the bathroom. The instructions weren't as clear as they could be. There's an exciting moment, after electrical DIY, when you switch on the appliance not knowing if it will work or blow up. It's a mixture of curiosity and responsibility similar to the opening night of a play. Tonight, it worked. I also attached two hooks to the bathroom wall so we can hang up the baby bath. Felt like a real man after all that.

Tomorrow is Kate's last day at work before beginning six months of maternity leave. This evening she went out for a few drinks with colleagues. She showed me what people have written in the Good Luck cards.

Alison, who hasn't got any kids, wrote: 'Enjoy the long-awaited & well-deserved rest.'

Cheryl, who has two kids, wrote more realistically: 'I wish you all the strength for the tough times and hope you enjoy the fantastic times!'

Friday 16 May
This time we didn't have to wait long before the squat midwife called Kate's name and ushered us into a room.

'Hello. How are you? Baby still inside? Ha ha ha.' She was one of those people who laugh at their own jokes. She had a big laugh and a toothy smile. 'My name is Audrey, by the way. Have we met before?'

In fact they met last week when Kate asked to see the senior midwife to complain about being kept waiting for nearly two hours. Audrey was the senior midwife.

'I'm not sure,' said Kate.

'I'm one of the midwives here,' said Audrey. 'In fact, I'm the only one here today.' Every midwife we've met has griped wryly about understaffing. 'Your blood pressure is fine. How are you feeling?'

'I've had a few twinges.'

'You don't want the baby to come early, do you? Ha ha ha.'

'No,' said Kate, 'I only finish work today.'

'Oh! Yes, you want a few days to be by yourself and spoil yourself for a while.'

We listened to the heartbeat, a swishing rhythm, like the rippling of a sheet of metal.

Audrey felt the bump and told us that the baby has partly engaged.

According to Audrey, the baby is lying on the right-hand side now. Ideally it should be on the left side. She said it doesn't make much difference. 'Unless the back is towards your back, that can be a little difficult. Keep active. Go for a walk each day. That will help things.'

She measured the bump and explained, 'The measurement has gone down a bit because there's more of the head in the pelvis. It is three-fifths palpable. Technically it hasn't officially engaged because the amount of the head above the pelvis is more than what's in the pelvis ... but it's getting there.'

She asked if we had any questions. Kate said, 'I have one slightly odd question. Should I be able to see the hole in my nipple where the milk comes out? Because I've looked and I can't see it.'

Audrey, who must've heard a million anxious questions from pregnant women, seemed to think this was one of the funniest. She emitted a toothy laugh. 'I'm sure it'll come out. Otherwise, if it doesn't, we'll stick a needle in. Ha ha ha.'

In the evening we went back to Herne Hill for an NCT class about the second stage of labour.

After the first stage of labour, when the cervix dilates, there is a transitional stage. This is when the woman might start screaming, shouting or biting. This peculiar behaviour tends to last for a few minutes or up to half an hour, 'then it calms down'.

The second stage, Jan says, 'is the best massage a baby will ever get'. It stimulates the baby's entire system and squeezes out a lot of mucus. A baby born by Caesarean misses out on the benefits of the journey along the vaginal canal, and the nurses and doctors need to compensate for this by manual stimulation and using suction to remove the mucus.

Jan warned us that squeezing through the narrow birth canal can elongate the baby's head. 'Some babies look shocking, freaky, like aliens.' It can be disturbing for the partner who is watching the baby emerge from the vagina. 'The partner sees a bit of head, then a bit more head, then a bit more head, then a bit more head, and he thinks, oh my God, how long is this baby's head?' But the distortion sorts itself out within hours or, more likely, days.

If everything is going well, the father can be there to 'catch the baby' as it comes out. 'But this should be discussed this with the medical team beforehand,' said Jan, 'don't just barge them out of the way at the last minute.'

Jan asked the men in the room if they wanted to cut the umbilical cord. Two or three of us did. The others weren't too keen. Gerry said nervously, 'Is it quite bloody?'

It's not very bloody, according to Jan. 'You can't go wrong. The midwife will give you a pair of rounded-edge scissors. You don't need to whip out a Swiss army knife or start gnawing through it. There are no nerves going through it so you won't hurt the baby or the mother. It's not one quick snip. It's a bit gristly.'

Lynne's husband still seemed to be worried about blood. 'Is there quite a lot of blood?'

Jan said, 'No, it's not like a butcher's shop.'

He seemed relieved. He had been concerned about getting it on his clothes. 'I was going to turn up in my painting gear.'

After tea and biscuits, Jan talked about the first hour after the birth. The mother might feel a rush of love for the baby, or she might not. She might feel emotionally flat. She might feel protective, but love might take longer. Jan said, 'Whatever your feelings, they're normal.'

If your baby needs to be taken to the special care unit, the father has a terrible dilemma. Go with the baby or stay with the mother? In practice, most mothers say, 'Don't let that baby out of your sight.' At this moment, the father's job is to do what he's told.

One in ten thousand babies haemorrhage. For this reason most hospitals give the baby an injection of vitamin K to encourage blood-clotting. Most parents let their baby receive the injection. Some parents prefer the vitamin K to be administered orally. Some forgo it altogether. There is vitamin K in colostrum, the substance produced from the mother's breasts in the first few days. The choice about vitamin K is the first choice you make for your baby. 'The first of many,' says Jan.

Jan began talking about the third stage, the delivery of the placenta. The word 'placenta' means 'flat cake' in Greek because it was believed that babies ate this cake in the womb.

I was sitting near Gerry, who had earlier admitted to feeling squeamish about the prospect of blood. He didn't seem keen on the idea of the placenta either. His eyes were rolling slowly. He was blinking a lot. He was squeezing his fingers.

If you've had a straightforward delivery, you can leave the placenta to come out in its own time. This usually takes between 30 to 40 minutes. 'Some people will tell you that, if you have a natural third stage, you'll bleed to death.' This is an exaggeration.

Newborns don't look like the immaculate babies in the nappy adverts. Jan showed us photos of some of the common distortions and blemishes. We saw cross-eyed, bruised, cone-headed, slimy, puffy-faced babies. We saw babies with peeling skin, rashes, swollen breasts, a swollen scrotum, a swollen labia, cold hands and a lip blister from sucking in the womb.

Finally, we asked Jan if it makes much difference if the baby is on the left side or the right side as it engages? We've heard conflicting opinions. Jan said, 'It doesn't make that much difference. I really wouldn't worry about it. Don't get paranoid.'

She told us all that one of the benefits of the NCT classes is that we can phone her for advice at any time during the next 18 years.

Kate felt 'quite a few' twinges all day. The baby was moving around a lot. 'I've got a feeling she's going to come soon.'

Towards midnight I was washing the dishes when Kate came into the kitchen, naked and smiling, showing me the bump. 'Look! It's huge!'

Saturday 17 May

I asked the baby not to be born today. It's the FA Cup final.

The baby's name is still supposed to be a secret. We use her name when we talk to her but not when other people are around. It's easy to blurt it out inadvertently. I did it today. Talking to a friend on the phone, I referred to the baby as Alice. He pretended not to notice.

Kate says that people at work have tried to trick her into revealing the baby's name. 'So what was her name again?' asked Debbie. Kate nearly fell into the trap.

Kate has bought a new diary. Her old diary, which she used for work, was 9 inches by 6 inches, a page a day, with the day divided into hours. Her new diary, for her new life on maternity leave, is about 3 inches by 2 inches; every day is a rectangular void and an entire week fits into 2 small pages.

While I was watching the football, Kate went to plant green beans on a hillside overlooking Dulwich. Weeks of antenatal yoga have barely alleviated the pains of gardening, never mind childbirth. When she came home she said, 'I've got stiff legs. If I'm like that after two hours on the allotment, what's labour going to be like?'

Feeling that I ought to say something encouraging, I said, 'Millions of women give birth every day.'

'I know. That doesn't help.'

We went to a barbecue in Clapham. In the bathroom, Kate weighed herself and was shocked. After that, she spent the rest of the party telling everyone that she weighs 81 kilos. Nearly 13 stone. People were smoking and Kate couldn't sit down because there weren't enough seats. We left early.

At home, Kate looked in the baby books. '"A woman can gain anything from almost nothing to 23 kilos",' she read. '"The average weight gain is 14 kilos."' Kate has gained 16 kilos.

Getting ready for bed, she grimaced. She has had twinges all day. They're just Braxton Hicks contractions, she thinks.

Our baby will be here soon. To have and to hold. In sickness and in health. For richer for poorer.

'It's gonna be amazing,' said Kate.

Sunday 18 May   **Week 40**

I slept really well. When I was ready to get up, I made myself stay in bed a bit longer, trying to memorise the feeling of lying in bed as long as I want after a good night's sleep.

'Oh, I had a terrible night,' said Kate.

'What with?'

'Heartburn. And I just felt like I was suffocating.' She had slept on the sofa for an hour and a half because there was more air in that room.

Sarah knows an obstetrician whose wife is having a baby. He has persuaded his wife to opt for an elective Caesarean 'because he's seen so many things go wrong in birth that he doesn't want to put his wife through that'. I haven't passed on this anecdote to Kate.

Not exactly an adventurous day. We went out twice. A trip to Sainsbury's. And a stroll around the block. When we got home after our walk, I had to help Kate up the stairs by pushing her from behind. At suppertime she put two thick telephone directories under her plate to make the food more reachable. She can't lean over her bump.

Kate worked all day and all evening, beyond midnight, writing reports for work. She wants to feel that she has completed all her admin.

She feels weighty in the pelvis. The baby hasn't moved so much today. 'I hope she's all right in there,' she fretted.

Monday 19 May

This was supposed to be her first day of maternity leave. Instead she went to work to finish some reports. Her caseload was so big that it has taken her a month just to bring all her paperwork up to date.

In the afternoon, being pregnant enabled her to evade a parking ticket. She had parked in front of Brixton Wholefoods. She was waiting to pay for an armful of cereal bars, which she plans to take to the labour ward as an emergency food supply, when a woman entered the shop warning people that there was a traffic warden outside. Kate waddled to the car just as the traffic warden was preparing a penalty notice. She pleaded her case. 'Oh please don't give me a ticket. I'm pregnant and I couldn't move fast enough.' This pathetic excuse seemed to work. The traffic warden stared at her blankly, but walked away without giving her a ticket.

Abigail, from our NCT group, phoned this afternoon to ask what kind of TENS machine is supposed to be best. I was able to tell her that the

802b is said to be more effective than the Lady TENS. My head is full of this kind of stuff.

Kate phoned me from work at 7.15 pm to say, 'I've finished. Everything.' She came home with a big smile on her face. All being well, she doesn't have to go back to work for eight months. She has six months of maternity leave. Three weeks of holiday. About a month of unpaid leave. And Christmas holidays.

After supper she said, 'What am I going to do tomorrow?'

She feels heavier since she weighed herself.

She feels as if she needs to sit with her legs apart. The baby is burrowing lower in the pelvis.

'It's weird,' said Kate, 'not knowing when it's going to happen.'

Tuesday 20 May

Kate's first day without work. After breakfast, she tidied the old suitcase where we keep all the tools. She prepared a lentil stew. She cleaned the bathroom sink. Still 'feeling at a loose end', she contemplated going for a swim at Dulwich Baths. Instead she decided to lie on the bed and read a book. In the afternoon she had a stroke of luck. A friend phoned wanting her advice about his son who needs the attentions of a psychologist. Kate was delighted. 'Something to do!' she joked. Then she went shopping for birthday presents for some relatives.

By late afternoon she looked dopey and was wandering aimlessly around the flat. 'I don't know what to do.'

Sometimes I only find out about her feelings by listening to what she tells her friends on the phone. Apparently her brain has started to disintegrate during the past two or three weeks. 'I haven't been able to do three things at once,' she told Elaine, 'and I've forgotten words just before I've got to them in a sentence.'

Kate told Elaine that she had a couple of months of regret about the effects pregnancy is going to have on her career. 'But I'm not bothered about that now.'

She told Elaine: 'I don't want to lose control. After a certain point, if it gets to induction and all that, it feels like it gets taken over by the medics and I just don't want that.'

She didn't even like it when she was obliged to ask a colleague at work to move a chair for her. 'It's frustrating,' she says, 'not being able to do things for myself.'

But the bump has forced her to overcome her reluctance to accept help. Which means I am becoming more useful. Increasingly, when she opens her mouth, the first thing she says is, 'Can you do me a favour?'

'I can feel numbness here,' she said, indicating both sides of her groin, 'waves of numbness as if something is pressing down.'

Wednesday 21 May

I still fear how I will react if our baby has Down's syndrome. There was a young lad with Down's syndrome on television this morning. I just thought: please, no, not that.

If it happens, I expect I will do the right thing, but I will feel the wrong thing. Disappointment. Revulsion.

I like to think that I'm a nice person but I appear to be a twat after all.

My mum has asked me to let her know when Kate goes into labour. She wants to be told as soon as the whole process starts. I know it's not a crime for a grandmother to want to see her grandchild. But I am feeling a rising sense of encroachment.

Kate and I discussed whether we want people around in the days after the birth. Kate thinks she will want to see people to share the 'excitement and amazement'. I would prefer it if everyone left us alone for six months.

Friends and family are phoning to ask how Kate is. People smile and squeal with enthusiasm when they see her. I feel like Scrooge. Because I don't feel undiluted joy. I'm feeling claustrophobic already at the thought of losing all my private time and space. I'm trying not to share these self-pitiful concerns with Kate. This isn't the time to appear miserable or doubtful. It's a birth, not a death. I must remember that. It's a good thing that's happening.

I'm not really worried about the practical aspects of childcare. I'm sure that, like everyone, we'll cope. What bothers me, periodically, is the psychological impact of losing so much private time and space.

I'm on a ride that I can't get off, whether I want to or not, and it lasts for the rest of my life.

'Are you excited?' People keep asking me this. My mum said it today.

'I am,' I replied, 'on the whole.'

'It'll be wonderful. You'll see.'

I'm still not totally convinced.

Parenthood is the biggest leap of faith an atheist can make.

I feel under pressure to be happy and excited. As if I'm not allowed to have mixed feelings.

I feel uneasy doing something that people approve of.

Kate was rather glum and grumpy and teary-eyed. She was worried because she hadn't felt the baby move much today. Late in the evening, there were a few kicks, and I listened to the heartbeat and reported that it was loud and regular. That cheered her up.

Thursday 22 May

Seven hours of sleep appears to have cured yesterday's bout of antenatal depression. Yesterday's anxiousness seems pathetic today.

Our final NCT class. Four hours discussing what happens after the birth.

'That's when it sinks in,' says Jan, 'when you leave the hospital and you're left alone with the baby.'

You might be quite tearful for a few days. Feeling 'up and down' at this stage is still normal.

Your baby's first bowel movement will produce a black and sticky substance called meconium. Spreading almond oil on your baby's bottom makes this easier to remove. While the baby is ingesting colostrum, the pooh is likely to be bright green. When it is living on full milk, the pooh is a mustardy yellow.

Don't panic if your baby loses weight in the days after birth. This is normal. 'It's a design feature,' says Jan.

We paused for lunch. As we gathered around the table, I was barged from behind by someone's bump. 'Sorry,' said Lynne, 'I keep doing that. I keep bumping into door frames.'

Abigail said she showed her bump to a friend. Her friend said, 'Gross!'

A couple of the women want their babies to come early 'before it gets too big'. One woman, Abigail, says that, as well as the *linea nigra*, she has a brown line on each of her breasts. 'I look like a zebra.'

'Most people are never shown how to bath their baby,' continues Jan. 'It's a bit nerve-wracking the first time.'

How to bath a baby? Jan recommended the little deckchairs that the baby can sit on. Or you can stand at the sink and wash the baby with water from a bowl. Even better, she says, is to get in the bath with your baby. Sit down, with your knees raised, and prop the baby on your legs where you can look at each other. It's nice for dads to do this. It's a bonding thing. If feeding is mainly mum-and-baby time, bathing can be dad-and-baby time.

Where should the baby sleep? It is strongly recommended that a baby sleeps in the same room as the parents for the first three to six months. A baby's breathing can be erratic. If a baby can hear an adult breathing, this helps to regulate its own breathing.

Babies are noisy sleepers. Jan warns us to expect 'farmyard noises'.

Kate says that she has noticed that she is 'more aware of birdsong early in the morning'. Jan says, 'Ah! That's preparing you for the baby.'

Hats are vital when you take a baby out of the house. Most of the baby's body heat is lost through the head. You can get nice hats in places like Baby Gap.

'A dangerous place to go,' said Abigail. 'It's too tempting.'

Jan warned us that the washing machine will be on several times a day. (This worries me. When our washing machine is on, the whole flat shakes. We'll be living in a giant washing machine.)

Jan produced a doll and asked us to pass it around the room, each holding the baby in a different position. One woman held the doll as if it was a bomb.

Finally Jan asked if our babies' grandparents would be coming to visit. There were conspicuous differences. Kate said that her mother-in-law might drive down from Manchester as soon as she hears that she has gone into labour. Another woman told us that her mother had said 'it was too far to come'.

'Where does your mother live?' asked Jan.

'North London,' said the woman. 'They don't like coming south of the river.'

Jan suggests that, if the grandparents come to visit, we should make it clear what their role is. Don't let them assume that they're expected, or allowed, to take over the childcare duties. One woman remembered practising for her driving test and being given advice by her mother that was years out of date. But her mother insisted that she was correct. So the woman did an emergency stop and showed her mother the Highway Code to prove who was right. 'And I know she'll be like that about the baby. If I let her.'

Jan encouraged us all to meet weekly in each other's houses.

In the beginning, all friendships are opportunistic. This is certainly true of friends made at parenting classes. It's useful to know people in the same boat, or at least afloat in the same sea, in the same storm.

'That's it,' said Jan. 'You're free to go.'

Kate's body keeps scaring her. Carrying a shopping bag from Peckham, her hand swelled to twice its normal thickness. She sat for ten minutes with both hands in the air, as if surrendering.

Friday 23 May
Kate says she should be entitled to more of the bed. Last night, I was too heavy to push away, so she poked me in the stomach until I moved. I don't remember that.

I do recall her stroking my arm at one point, to reassure me of her affection, before she immediately tried to shove me further towards the wall.

The antenatal appointments at the hospital are weekly now. 'You've had a lot of appointments, haven't you?' said the midwife, Andrea. She is the one with the frozen face. When she tries to smile, her features don't move. 'I suppose you just come when you're told, don't you? According to studies, the optimal number of appointments is four.'

Kate asked what the average number of antenatal appointments is at this hospital.

'Six or seven,' said Andrea. 'I don't think people would feel happy with any less. Things can change quickly. How are you?'

Kate said that she has been feeling an extra weightiness, not constantly, just for half an hour at a time, as if the baby is burrowing down. She has only felt five or six minor contractions over the past week.

'It varies so much with different people,' said Andrea. 'Some people feel contractions for weeks on end.'

Blood pressure normal. Urine normal.

Andrea said, 'Are you managing to get some rest, as much as you can?' Last week a different midwife told her to go for regular walks.

Andrea felt the bump and declared it three-fifths palpable, meaning that most of the baby's head still hasn't engaged.

The heartbeat 'sounds good'.

We have another appointment next Friday. If the baby hasn't arrived by then, Andrea suggested, someone might do 'a sweep'. A doctor will 'run a finger around the neck of the womb' to stimulate the production of prostaglandin. It's uncomfortable but not painful, she said.

Outside, waiting to cross the road, Kate stood close to me. 'Maybe we can do our own sweep instead. With your willy.'

Now she's interested.

Yet another trip to Herne Hill for a NCT class. We were joining another group for a couple of hours to make up for the class we missed when we were at a wedding. Eight women and five men. We recognised three couples from the NHS classes. Belt and braces people, like us.

One of the first signs of labour, says Jan, is the nesting instinct. One man came home to find his wife vacuuming his toolbox and polishing his saw. She had already cleaned everything else in the house. Jan said, 'Don't be surprised if you wake up in the middle of the night with a desire to start scrubbing things. When I had my second baby, I cleaned the kitchen ceiling at two o'clock in the morning.'

About 20 per cent of women experience their waters breaking in the two or three days before labour. It can be a gradual trickle or a massive gush. It is most likely to occur at night when the hormones are most active. In Jan's case, she heard a loud pop and 2 litres of water poured out. It's a good idea to protect your mattress with plastic sheeting or a bin bag.

When the contractions begin, try to keep calm. Eat well. Pasta. Bread. Sandwiches. Mashed potatoes. Food for a marathon.

Distract yourself with dull videos. Get some fresh air if it's a nice day. Be careful about phoning people. Unless you want them getting overexcited and turning up at the hospital. Some people do that.

As soon as labour starts, partners should try to be present and available. A woman in labour wants to feel that someone is around, that she isn't alone.

You might feel so comfortable in the bath that you don't want to get out. But, in early labour, you're not supposed to stay in a bath for more than 15–20 minutes. It can slow or stop contractions. So don't be tempted to lie in the bath. 'This is D-Day,' said Jan, 'time to get the baby out.'

You shouldn't go into hospital until your contractions are occurring every 3–4 minutes and lasting 40–50 seconds. The length of the contractions is as important as the frequency.

Most women find the journey to hospital really difficult. Usually they travel on all fours on the back seat. It's stressful for the driver too, listening to a howling woman complaining about every bump in the road. 'It's not the easiest journey, but somehow you'll do it.'

In the hospital, you'll be given an internal examination to estimate how dilated you are. The midwife will measure your cervix with her fingers. Three centimetres of dilation is roughly equal to the width of two fingers. The midwife may ask you to lie on your back for this examination. You might not like the idea of this. You can ask to be examined in an upright position, even if this is more awkward for the midwife.

These days the most common method of monitoring the baby during labour is with a handheld sonic aid. If for some reason they decide to use a foetal belt monitor, remember that this requires you to keep still for a considerable time, so make sure you're in a comfortable, sustainable position before they strap the belt on. You might find that lying on your back puts too much pressure on your lower spine. This is the moment where your partner needs to be assertive on your behalf, because you might be feeling too vulnerable to state your preferences.

You're not ill. This is a positive thing that's happening. Get the bed pushed to the side of the room if you want more space. Put a beanbag or a mat or a birthing ball on the floor – anything that helps you to create a personal nest, a cosy corner. This is what all animals do when they're giving birth. They need to feel safe and content with the environment or the labour doesn't progress. It's not unknown for contractions to stop if the woman is dissatisfied with the space.

'If you're not happy with the midwife,' said Jan, 'ask for a new one. Speak to the supervisor. It's very likely that if you don't like her, she won't like you either.'

Students can be enthusiastic and helpful during a labour, but don't allow more than one in the room. If there are two or more, they tend to spend the time chatting to each other.

Your contractions should build until they are lasting for 1–2 minutes and are only 30 seconds apart. This phase can 'kick in' anytime from the point that you're 5–6 centimetres dilated.

Many women say that the most difficult part is getting from 6 centimetres to 10 centimetres. On average, for a first birth, the cervix dilates at a rate of 1 centimetre per hour. But there are wide variations.

At 9 or 10 centimetres, you reach 'the point where you lose the plot'. Some women become verbally or physically abusive, swearing and scratching. Make sure that you've cut your fingernails.

Much of the abuse is aimed at the partner. This isn't the moment to take offence. 'It's not the time to say, "If that's your attitude, I'm off."'

This transition stage can last for a few minutes or for half an hour. You might feel sick and shivery. Have a blanket or a dressing gown handy to keep you warm.

Make the V-sign with two fingers. The distance between your fingertips is as wide as your cervix needs to be when it's fully dilated.

Getting from 3 centimetres to 10 centimetres takes 15 hours on average. But it could be much quicker. Or it could take two or three days.

Some of the women in the group have been told by midwives that they don't need a birth plan. Jan says they're wrong.

Jan demonstrated that a cushion on top of a bucket makes a comfortable seat for a pregnant woman, reducing the pressure on the spinal column.

On the way home, we bought a bucket.

That's the last of the classes. The days are mine again.

In the afternoon I had work to do. Instead I assembled the rocking frame for the carrycot, fitted sunshades to the car windows and installed the car seat. Kate was lying on the bed so I cuddled behind her. I was just drifting towards sleep when she rolled over and I saw that she was crying.

This is one of the duties of intimacy. You have to show love and tenderness when you don't feel loving or tender. I just felt tired and perplexed and frustrated. I hugged her and stroked her hair. During a brief lull between the spasms of tears, I asked why she was crying.

'I feel lonely,' she said.

I felt bad. It's my fault. I'm poor company when I'm working, and I've been working a lot. Normally I try to wait until she's at work or in bed before sitting at my desk. But now she is at home all the time. She feels excluded and I feel intruded upon; she feels lonely and I feel claustrophobic.

These are big changes we'll have to get used to.

Saturday 24 May

Kate feels that she has got fatter in the past couple of weeks. She makes the floorboards in the bathroom creak.

We spoke on the phone to a friend whose baby is less than a year old. She told us ominously, 'Make the most of your time together.'

It's impossible to reconcile all the competing demands. To rest. To spend time together. To work hard while I still have the hours and the energy.

Today, realising that my working habits have become frantic and asocial, I forced myself to put work to one side.

When we woke up the sun was shining so we discussed going to a park, although Kate was worried that she wouldn't be able to walk for long. By the time we were ready to leave the flat, there were charcoal clouds, so instead of strolling on Hampstead Heath, we went shopping in central London. This probably isn't the best thing to do on the day before you're due to give birth. The streets were hectic. It was like Piccadilly Circus. In fact, it was Piccadilly Circus. And Tottenham Court Road. And Oxford Street. We spent the afternoon in Habitat and John Lewis, looking for things that weren't there.

Since scrupulously making lists of things to buy and things to do, I've been reluctant to go near them, as if the shopping lists are quicksand. Today I plunged in and went hunting for a few essential items that I still need for the birth. One of them was a black and white film for my camera. So we went to Jessops, the photography shop on New Oxford Street. Black and white films are sold in the basement, down a steep flight of steps, so Kate stayed upstairs. When I returned, she was buying a digital camera costing £244. The teenage salesman was trying to promote the compact camera to his pregnant client by telling her that 'it's good for taking pictures at parties'.

Kate wants to email our baby to her relatives in France. That's fine, except that it has caused us to spend £244 when we only went into the shop to buy a roll of film. Afterwards we invented a rule. In future we won't make impulse purchases costing more than £50.

I keep forgetting, and walk too fast. We ended up traipsing further than we'd anticipated. The energy expended on Oxford Street could've fuelled three circuits of Hampstead Heath. In a department store, she rested on a rocking chair with a rocking footstool. I lay in a hammock. Then I went to fetch the car while she sat on a bench in a park behind John Lewis. 'Too much,' said Kate.

Sunday 25 May   **Due Date**   **Week** 41

Last week, a good friend phoned and asked, 'What are you doing on Sunday?'

'Having a baby.'

'Apart from that.'

'Nothing.'

'Shall I come round in the afternoon?'

'OK.'

A while ago, someone advised us to arrange a social event for the evening of the due date. A trip to a cinema or a restaurant. Anything that distracts you from the non-appearance of your baby.

So our friend came round, having phoned first to ensure that it was safe. When he arrived, I told him the bad news. I would be cooking.

'Pasta?' he guessed cynically, knowing my limits. 'You'd better hope your baby likes pasta.'

Cheeky bastard. As it happened, it was pasta.

A lot of women are bored of being pregnant by this stage. Kate says that she isn't bored. But she wants to hold the baby and know that she is well. So she wants the baby to come out now.

When people phone up and ask what we're doing, I say, 'Just waiting.' But I'm not just waiting. I'm working manically, while I can.

The bump is bigger and longer. It is a zeppelin. Increasingly, Kate has trouble breathing. Drying herself after a bath, patting and panting, trying to reach the furthest regions of her body, she sounds as if she's walking uphill.

I opened the bedroom door and found her massaging her perineum and frowning. 'I don't think this is doing any good,' she said.

'Well ...' I tried to think of a reassuring argument. 'Just try to relax, lovey.'

'It's going to be painful.'

'It will be, but it's a temporary pain, and we'll have our baby as a reward.'

'I keep having morbid thoughts.'

'It'll be fine. You've got a strong, healthy body. You've been eating all the right things. Doing lots of exercise. I just think she'll be fine.'

It is past midnight now. Our baby is not one of the 4 per cent born on the due day. She has at least one thing in common with her father – she misses deadlines.

No show.

Monday 26 May

Apparently, Kate got out of bed for an hour during the night, unable to sleep because of heartburn. I slept through everything.

Now she is fed up. In the afternoon, returning from lunch at a friend's house, she realised that her diary is entirely blank. Bereft of work and social engagements, she is just waiting. After an hour of this void, she admitted, 'I'm starting to get bored.'

We strolled around Dulwich Park in the sunshine. She can walk or talk, but she can't do both at the same time. Her lungs can't muster enough breath.

I practised carrying the stuff that we want to take into the hospital. I will have to carry a large backpack, two shoulder bags, a bucket and a giant birthing ball.

When she stopped laughing, Kate took a photo of me weighed down under all the stuff. I imagined our daughter looking at this photo, of her dad as a mule, in an album many years from now. It was the first time I've had to arrange my face knowing that my daughter was looking at me. So I smiled benignly at the camera for her, pleased to be able to communicate at last.

I talk to the baby every night, and I listen to her heartbeat. But we're keen to hold her now and get to know her properly. I have a suspicion that parenthood is much more satisfying than pregnancy. Well, we're about to find out.

Harriet phoned from Yorkshire, hoping that our baby had been born today, on Kate's brother's birthday. There are several shared birthdays in Kate's family. It gives her granny fewer dates to remember.

Kate has been feeling slight period pains. Knowing that this is one of the first indications that labour is beginning, we felt excited and apprehensive, until she read in a book that these pains can last for several days.

Kate is starting to worry that the doctors will want to induce the birth. She is so desperate to avoid this; she even talked about the possibility of having sex to initiate the labour. It was one of those rare occasions when I found myself arguing against the idea. She has been feeling so delicate and protective in that area, I just know that we would have to abort the mission.

Also, the baby is conspicuous by her presence now; it would be like having sex with a baby between us.

I have no rational reason for thinking this, but I just believe that everything will be OK.

Tuesday 27 May

Kate slept soundly, but not soundlessly. She snored like a pot-bellied pig.

Her aunt phoned to ask if she is still 'a lady in waiting'. Delighted to have something to do, Kate went to visit her aunt and cousin in Pimlico. She sat on a towel in the car. When she got home, she reported no new feelings. 'Just the same. Kind of period painy.'

A friend, Phil, assures me that he also went to hospital with 101 bags when his wife was pregnant. He also felt a fool. This evening I was given permission to play football as long as I checked my phone regularly during the game.

'Will you look at my vagina?'

I looked at it.

'Is it swollen? Is it red?'

I wasn't much help. I said, 'The truth is, I can't remember what it used to be like, it's been so long since I've seen it.'

Kate's dad, who never gets in touch, has been in touch. She checked her email for the first time in a while and found a message from him, sent on her due date, asking for news and saying he was 'thinking about her a lot'.

Wednesday 28 May

When I finally forced myself out of bed, I found a card on my desk. It had hearts on the front. Inside she had written:

> My love,
>
> Happy Anniversary, I love you very much and even though things will change with baby we must always make sure we make time for us.
>
> I love you xxxx'

I was moved. A powerful emotion stirred within me. It was a feeling of panic. I'd forgotten to get her a card. I quietly retired to the bedroom where I keep a few miscellaneous cards in a box under the bed. Birthday cards. Thank You cards. All useless. Then I was lucky. I found a card featuring two lovers, tête-à-tête, making eyes at each other. One of the lovers was Elmer, the multicoloured patchwork elephant, and the other lover was Elmer's black-and-white elephant friend, Wilbur. I gave it to Kate and she seemed pleased.

Later in the day she said, 'The card you gave me for Mother's Day had an elephant on it as well. Are you trying to tell me something?'

I wasn't. We saw elephants when we were in Nepal. That's all I meant by it.

She feels like Elmer. 'God, I'm fat,' she said, stepping back to see herself in the mirror. 'My arms have gone fat.'

On a whim, we went to Brighton for the day. We went there exactly four years ago on our first date, cycling along the seafront and over the South Downs. This time we were less energetic. In the car, Kate sat on a towel.

The sea was flat and calm but the air trembled with the heat.

Women who aren't pregnant look weird. I saw a woman running in a bikini. I was shocked to see her flat stomach and a body shaped like an hourglass rather than a pint glass. It fascinated me as much as Kate's belly fascinates non-pregnant people.

She wanted to go to the water's edge but didn't think she'd be able to climb back up the slope of the beach over the shingle. She felt stranded, like a whale. 'I feel a bit beached.'

We drove along the coast into Brighton and walked around the Lanes, feeling as if we were on holiday. I saw Kate frowning at a shop window. I said, 'What are you looking at?'

'Myself,' she said. 'I keep shocking myself, in all these shop windows.'

We sat on Brighton beach and ate fish and chips because we liked the idea of it. At dusk, heading home, we parked on the South Downs and sat on a hill with a flask of tea and Kate's home-made chocolate brownies. The sun, low and red, with a wisp of cloud in front of it, looked like Saturn.

Back home, she felt sick. Nausea at this stage can be a sign of labour. It can also be a sign of greasy food. 'I wish I hadn't eaten the fish and chips,' she said sorrowfully.

Before we went to bed, she said, 'I think it might be tonight we go to the hospital. I've got strong period pains.'

Call it feminine intuition. Call it a mother's instinct. Whatever it was, it was wrong. We had a peaceful night.

Thursday 29 May

This morning in bed, her chat-up line was unusual. 'I want your prostaglandin.' Prostaglandin, the chemical that initiates labour, is also found in sperm.

Suddenly she wasn't feeling so fragile down there. I tried not to think about the other person in bed with us. It was slightly awkward, as if we were trying to dance the tango for the first time in years, with a baby squashed between us. At times it was as erotic as fitting a washing machine. Despite the obstacles to pleasure, she said her orgasm was 'amazing' – but the first one in three months tends to be.

Kate is still acclimatising herself to being at home all the time. She isn't used to having empty days. She pottered around the flat, trying on hats.

Her only appointment of the day was cancelled. She had arranged to meet socially with the other pregnant women from the NCT classes – one of the aims of the NCT is to encourage women to form 'self-supporting groups'. Today's meeting was supposed to be at Rita's house, but Rita phoned this morning to say that she has diarrhoea and vomiting. Pregnancy makes strangers feel able to share these details.

A friend phoned and invited us to a comedy club in Bethnal Green this evening. She said it would take our mind off things. We imagined sitting in a smoky room watching other people get drunk. In the end we opted for less boisterous pleasures, more in keeping with our age and status: we went to Nunhead Cemetery and sat on a bench. There's a fine view of St Paul's from the hill. But the wooden slats were hard. So we relocated to grassy Peckham Rye where we found a tree to lie under. 'This is what I wanted!' said Kate, arranging herself with her head in the shade and her body in the sunshine.

In the evening I cycled to the hospital to check where I can park the car. We have an antenatal appointment in the morning. The midwife has suggested that they might perform 'a sweep' of the cervix. Kate has been worrying about this and none of the books mention it, so she phoned Jan, the NCT teacher, for information. Jan said that it's a fairly standard procedure to ascertain if the cervix is dilating and softening. The midwife squeezes her finger into the neck of the womb, if it's dilated enough, and runs a finger around the walls of the cervix, hoping that this will stimulate the release of prostaglandin. This is only possible if the cervix has begun to soften. Jan has heard that it's quite painful, which isn't what the midwife told us last week.

Kate told me that she has been having some morbid thoughts and was wondering if this is just normal anxiety or a kind of 'female intuition' that something is wrong. So I reminded her that female intuition told her that the labour was going to start last night. She asked me to listen to the baby's heart. It was loud and regular as always.

I'm not as worried as Kate is. A few days ago I stopped working so frantically, finally accepting that I won't be able to write eight plays and four novels before the baby is born, and since then I've been more relaxed about everything, enjoying the days more, and better company for Kate. John Wesley wrote: 'Beware you be not swallowed up in books! An ounce of love is worth a pound of knowledge.' I've finally got the message.

Friends are still phoning. Some of them are getting impatient.

We just have to live with this strange knowledge that our life is going to be turned upside down any day now. But which day?

Friday 30 May
It was a different midwife. This one was called Deirdre. Kate explained that she has been feeling period-type pains around her abdomen for a few days, and she can feel a weight on her perineum, especially at night.

'So,' said Deirdre, 'things are starting to happen slowly? That's fine.'

Kate said that she's been worried that the baby isn't moving enough. But when she described the movements, Deirdre seemed satisfied. 'As long as you're feeling at least ten per day,' she said. 'If you're anxious about it, take a day to write down every time you feel a movement, and you'll probably find it's 20 or 30 times.'

Last night, after talking about it, we decided to delay the sweep for a few days. Kate said, 'I don't want them sticking their fingers up there before they have to.'

So Kate raised the subject. Unlike last week's midwife, Deirdre didn't seem to think it was necessary yet. 'If you haven't given birth this time next week,' she said, 'you'll have to see a doctor who might do a sweep then.' There may also be another routine scan to check the baby. After that, they'll start thinking about induction. 'Are you happy to be induced?' asked Deirdre.

'I'd rather not,' said Kate.

'That's also another option,' said Deirdre. She wasn't discouraging. 'If you want to hang on for as long as possible. But at some point ...'

'I know.'

Kate's blood pressure was up, but within the normal limits. 'It tends to rise slightly at the end of pregnancy anyway.' The baby's heartbeat was normal.

Deirdre measured the bump. This number hasn't increased for the past few weeks. Naturally we fear that this is because the baby has stopped growing; it is dead and shrivelling. In fact, it's simply because there's less of the baby to measure. 'It feels like the head is quite deeply engaged,' said Deirdre. She wrote 'two-fifths palpable' on the medical notes. Which means three-fifths of the head is in the pelvis.

'You know there are other ways of speeding things along?' said Deirdre.

'Yes,' said Kate.

'Sex,' said Deirdre, making her point clear. She glanced at me. I wasn't sure what reaction was required from me. A wink? A leer? Gratitude? Something to confirm that the message had been received? *Roger, will do.* Maybe she was assessing me to see if I was up to the job.

'Or raspberry leaf tea,' said Deirdre.

Before we left, she turned to me again. 'Have you been given one of these?'

'No. Thank you.' It was glossy propaganda called *DAD* – 'the magazine for new fathers'. The cover photo was of Pierce Brosnan, the actor who plays

James Bond, who has five children. The headline promised: 'JAMES BOND'S TIPS FOR FATHERHOOD'. Another cover story was 'DAVID BECKHAM ON WHY FATHERHOOD IS MORE IMPORTANT THAN FOOTBALL'.

I read the magazine when I got home. Most of the adverts were selling designer clothes. An article promoting breastfeeding was illustrated by a photo of a sexy, naked female torso without a baby in sight – presumably to stop men flicking over the page. The magazine seemed to be aimed at a stereotypical male reader, obsessed with sex and football. I enjoyed it.

An article about post-natal sex advises men to write this phrase down and stick it up on a wall where you can see it every day before the baby comes: YOUR SEX LIFE WILL NEVER BE THE SAME AGAIN.

Elsewhere, a midwife writes that 'A man doesn't need to do much during labour, just being there – having your smell and voice there is virtually enough.' She makes it sound as if my physical presence is unnecessary. I can just send Kate into the labour ward with a tape of my voice and one of my unwashed T-shirts. This midwife advises men to says things like: 'You're doing brilliantly, darling, you brave woman.' I said this to Kate – she was stranded on the toilet trying to pooh – and she just laughed.

Kate is getting bored. She arranged a twilight barbecue on our allotment on Sydenham Hill. She phoned friends to invite them along. She wrote a list of the food. She selected the food in Sainsbury's. She unpacked the bags after I'd carried them inside. She is learning the art of making a simple task last all day.

One friend calls the baby The Wee One and she calls Kate The Fat One. 'How's the wee one? And how's the fat one?'

Kate needed to get home quickly for the loo. When she got there, nothing would come out. We tried to remember what we were told about pooh during the birthing classes. We couldn't remember. 'It's all confusion,' said Kate. 'Diarrhoea, pooh, show, waters …'

She is worrying all day now. Anxiety colours the background even when something else occupies the foreground of our attention. At bedtime, she was gloomy again. 'She isn't moving very much. I've been counting. I've counted four. Since this morning.'

I listened to the heartbeat. It was fast, regular, normal. As we were falling asleep, I could feel the baby's hiccups.

Saturday 31 May

Temperature of 28°C in the bedroom. Bikinis on Peckham Rye. We did a circuit of the whole park. One old lady saw Kate and said, 'I commiserate with you, dear.'

'I don't mind it,' said Kate, thinking the old lady was talking about the heat, but afterwards she wondered if the old lady was referring to her size and weight.

The baby has moved a lot today.

Kate wants the baby to come out. 'It's stressful. Aren't you stressed? You don't seem to be.'

I'm not stressed about that. I'll be pleased when the baby comes. I hope. Until then, I intend to enjoy every unfettered day and every sleep-drenched night.

In France, Kate says, a baby isn't regarded as full term until 41 weeks have passed. So, if we were living across the Channel, we wouldn't even be under this pressure to deliver.

Morbid thoughts. What if one of them died? What if they both died? Pregnancy is a marathon in which the sight of the finishing line brings no relief because the greatest obstacle and adversity is waiting there.

Sunday 1 June   **Week 42**

Woke up at 6.40 am when Kate called me to the loo to look at a piece of toilet paper. She held it up towards me. Saturated with the fluid that was seeping out of her, the tissue was pale brown with blood. There was a tiny clump of clear jelly. This was a show, the release of the mucus plug that seals the cervix during pregnancy and detaches as the cervix begins to open.

The books say a show might be 'blood-tinged' or 'blood-stained'. She was worried that there was more blood than there ought to be. I didn't know. So she phoned the labour ward at King's. The midwife told her to come in for an examination.

All my conscientious planning of the route was a waste of time. There were roadworks near the hospital. Signs directed us the wrong way down one-way streets.

We took the lift to the fourth floor where a midwife, a short West Indian woman, ushered us into one of the labour rooms. Without getting too close to it, she looked at the brown-stained toilet paper, which Kate had brought with her in a plastic bag. The midwife said it looked normal.

'What number baby is this?'

'Sorry?'

'Is this your first baby?'

'Yes,' said Kate.

The midwife checked Kate's temperature, blood pressure and urine. Everything was normal.

Around us, the rooms of labour ward were reassuringly silent.

'It's quiet today,' said Kate.

'It's not quiet,' said the midwife. 'There's no screaming, but it's not quiet.'

Kate lay on a bed, tilted at 45 degrees, while the midwife strapped two monitors around her stomach. One measured the baby's heartbeat. A squiggle of lines appeared on the graph paper spooling out of the machine next to the bed. We could hear the amplified heart, a steady drumbeat, like an army just over the hill.

The other monitor also produced a spool of graph paper. 'Oooh!' said the midwife when she saw the lines on the graph. 'Pain!'

'What?' said Kate.

'Did you feel that pain?'

'No.'

'The monitor shows uterine activity.'

We all looked. There were seismic contractions occurring every 1½ inches on the graph paper.

'Can't you feel that?' said the midwife.

'I can feel a kind of vague period pain,' said Kate doubtfully.

'That's a contraction,' said the midwife.

We have heard about women – extremely rare and fortunate women – who go through the whole process of childbirth experiencing only moderate discomfort rather than pain. Is Kate one of these rare, lucky women?

No, as it turns out, she isn't.

We were left alone in the room for 30 minutes. Kate was aware of the contractions now that they'd been pointed out to her. Each one felt like a long build-up of tension inside her abdomen, accompanied by a brief increase in the baby's heart rate.

We read novels while we waited for the doctor to appear. Kate nibbled a flapjack she'd brought from home. It was all very calm and civilised, like giving birth in the café at Books Etc.

The small West Indian midwife ended her shift and was replaced by a small Chinese midwife. When the doctor came, she was Indian. This is a rainbow hospital.

The doctor was going to examine Kate's cervix with a speculum, but changed her mind when it became apparent that Kate was producing no more blood or discharge. We were left alone again while they wrote a report in Kate's medical notes. Standing in the corridor, we watched the traffic of midwives and cleaners. Everyone smiled when they saw us.

Then the doctor came back. She had changed her mind. 'I don't feel happy,' she said, 'letting you go home without examining you.' So Kate lay back on the bed with her trousers down. They smile even when they're sticking a finger in your private parts. The doctor seemed content with what she found there. The cervix was still closed, but was softening.

Back home we went to bed and slept until the afternoon. Friends got excited when we didn't answer the phone. They left agitated messages, thinking we were giving birth, not realising that we were just asleep.

After breakfast at 2 pm Kate said, 'What shall I do?'

I told her to relax while she still had all this time to herself. But she was uncomfortable because of the period-type pains across her abdomen. She didn't want a bath. She didn't want to go for a walk. She went back to bed with a magazine.

'I'm in quite a lot of pain now,' she said. 'Well, not pain. I'm aware of it now.' We decided that it was time for the TENS machine. To be effective, it has to be attached before the labour pains become intense. Now seemed a good moment. I placed the four sticky pads on her back. Then I pulled them off and repositioned them.

'Are they in the right place?' she asked, as if she didn't trust me.

'Yes,' I said. I was fairly sure.

Even her dad phoned. It was the first time he'd called for years. It wasn't a long conversation but he concluded by saying, 'Love you, darling.' Which pleased her.

We weren't sure how quickly things would progress. Kate has read some unsettling stories about frighteningly quick labours. But the afternoon passed without a dramatic intensification of the contractions.

In the early evening we went to our friends' house in Brixton for tea and cakes. The idea was to take our mind off these early labour pains, but they were the principle topic of conversation.

Instead of driving straight home afterwards, we decided to go for a slow stroll around Myatt's Fields. A jogger completed ten circuits of the park for our one. Suddenly the contractions were only a few minutes apart, not quite regular, each lasting 10–30 seconds. It was time to go home.

I was excited now. The waiting was over. I was wearing a white shirt. I changed into a darker colour. Whatever lay ahead, I expected it to be messy.

I said to her, 'You're doing brilliantly, darling, you brave woman.' She laughed.

She phoned her brother and sister-in-law to tell them that things were starting to happen.

At 10 pm, both feeling excited, we went for a walk around the block. The romantic mood was slightly tarnished on Oglander Road when Kate stepped on a giant dog turd. 'Squeeze my hand,' I said when her pain came. She said I was squeezing her hand too hard.

On Bellenden Road we went to see the old junk shop that has been converted into a restaurant. As we examined the menu stuck on the window, the owner came outside to talk to us. He was quite tipsy. He admired Kate's bump. 'I've got three kids,' he said. 'It's the most wonderful thing.' He also claimed that he used to be a qualified midwife.

'When's it due?' he asked.

'Now,' I said. 'We're counting contractions.' He seemed momentarily taken aback, as if his midwifery skills might be called upon. It was an excuse to kiss Kate on the cheek. I didn't even get a handshake. He promised us 'a meal on the house'. As an afterthought he added, '… but you'll have to pay for the drinks.'

After a hot and wet day, the evening was warm and dry. We carried on walking along the neighbourhood's quieter, darker streets. 'Walking is helping,' said Kate. 'Maybe I'll just walk through the entire labour.' But then she decided it was time to go home. I was carrying my mobile phone because it had a stopwatch on it. By now the contractions were 3–6 minutes apart, each lasting 40 seconds, and getting progressively stronger. A midwife this morning told us to come into the hospital when they were 'three in ten'. Three contractions in ten minutes.

At home we phoned our mums to tell them that things were happening at last.

At 11.10 pm, Kate said 'Ow!' for the first time.

My tooth was aching. I've been having trouble with it for a couple of weeks but I've been delaying treatment until after the birth. Sod's law means that it has to get worse now. But it didn't seem the moment to complain to Kate.

I made food. Sweetcorn and pasta. During the contractions we had to stop eating so that she could stand up and lean on me. They were painful now – 5 minutes apart, each lasting about 35 seconds. At midnight she turned up the power on the TENS machine.

Monday 2 June

We were facing each other; she leant on me. She told me to lay my hands on her lower back and press so that she could push against them.

We watched a video. *Driving Miss Daisy*. It's a test of a good film if you can watch it while having contractions.

She tried changing position. She tried resting on the large blue birthing ball. She tried rocking to and fro.

By 2 am I was tired. I packed a bag with ham sandwiches and a flask of tea. I could see the advantages of having two birthing partners. Somebody else would be handy, so I could concentrate on Kate rather than on the sandwiches.

I was still using the stopwatch on my mobile phone to time the contractions. 'Now!' she said and I hurried to press the button that started the timer. Sometimes the contraction began and I forgot to press the button. At the end she said, 'How long was that one?' I made up an answer, inventing a figure that was plausible and encouraging, rather than demoralise her by admitting that I hadn't timed that one properly.

She lay on the bed. She lay on cushions on the floor. When the contractions came, she stood up and leant on me. 'You're doing well, you're doing well,' I kept saying. 'Remember it's for Alice.'

'Yeah.'

At 3.30 am we were listening to Eva Cassidy songs. I couldn't do anything for more than three or four minutes at a time. I rushed over whenever a contraction started. Massaging, rubbing, holding or just being leant on.

Outside there was a heavy, dramatic, pulverising rainstorm. The air was cooler. I put more clothes on.

When the contractions were 4 to 5 minutes apart and each lasting 50 seconds, Kate said she wanted to go to the hospital. I phoned the maternity ward and told the midwife on duty that we were on our way. I told her that we wanted to use the birthing pool.

At 4 am there are more foxes on the road than cars. I was halfway to the hospital when a car flashed its lights at me. I had forgotten to turn my headlights on.

I drove into the car park and chose the space nearest to the maternity building. Carrying all the bags, I lurched up the steps, along the foyer, into the lift, out of the lift and along the corridor to the maternity unit.

At reception we met the midwife I had spoken to on the phone. She did not inspire confidence. Nothing had been done to prepare for our arrival. They hadn't started filling the birthing pool. They hadn't even allocated us a room. She said that she was looking for a room for us. But most of the rooms were unoccupied.

The midwife told us to go to the waiting room. She indicated a room at the end of the corridor. The door was open. A man was in there. Kate decided to stand in the corridor instead. She didn't fancy having contractions in a public waiting room next to a stranger.

We had been told during previous visits to the maternity unit that there was a mobile birthing pool. Now the midwife was insisting that it wasn't available. It was lying unused in a room where a woman was giving birth. Instead the midwife wanted us to use a room with a built-in birthing pool but no natural light and stacks of furniture; we didn't like the idea of giving birth in a storeroom, so we asked if another room was available. She took us to room six, then redirected us to room nine.

I was carrying all the bags between the rooms. This meant I had to leave Kate alone for a couple of minutes. I was hauling the bags into our new room when Kate appeared in the corridor, her face full of tears. Some yards behind her, the midwife had an expression that I couldn't quite interpret. Later I realised that the look on her face was disguised guilt, culpability.

My first thought was that Kate was crying because of the pain and anxiety of the labour. It was only later that Kate told me what had happened while I was fetching and carrying the bags. The midwife had tried to dissuade her from using the birthing pool, especially when Kate mentioned that she only intended to use it for the labour but not the actual birth. The midwife seemed to find it too much trouble. 'Why use the birthing pool if you're not going to give birth in it?' the midwife said.

'Why don't you just have a bath?' This was the worst possible welcome to the hospital. Kate felt that she was being subtly bullied. This hospital goes to a lot of effort to promote birthing pools; bizarrely, when you turn up and ask for one, they try to talk you out of it while you're having contractions.

Eventually the midwife examined the dilation of the cervix and attached a belt to Kate's stomach for 20 minutes of foetal monitoring. Kate's contractions, which at home had been increasingly powerful and frequent, now diminished and stopped. Her body had shut down.

Kate's cervix wasn't dilated at all. The cervix was still posterior. Normally we'd be sent home, said the midwife. But we didn't fancy returning home with all our luggage and having to go through the whole journey again. We were allowed to stay. At the time we were pleased about this. Only later did we realise what a big mistake it was.

Kate asked me to wash the bath and the toilet in our room. She tried to relax in a warm bath. I sprayed her face and legs with cold water.

I had a sense of anticlimax. Tedium. Disappointment at the loss of momentum.

Kate reattached the TENS machine and walked around the room. The walls were white and pale blue. The armchair and the birthing ball were green. The bed and all the machinery were grey metal. As she paced up and down, she laughed. 'I feel like a prisoner,' she said.

The midwife returned. 'My name is Faith,' she said. I asked if there was a midwife experienced in water births. 'I am,' she said. My heart sank.

We watched Faith bickering with a junior midwife. It didn't inspire confidence.

For relaxation, Kate wanted Eva Cassidy and a bottom massage.

At 7 am, we ate some of the ham sandwiches. I drank peppermint tea from the flask.

The contractions began again.

'I'm wondering if we should go home,' said Kate. But we didn't.

'I wish you'd doze,' said Kate. 'It would make me feel something was going to happen.'

I was tired. Constantly getting up and down. She wanted me to doze but I had a lot to do. Getting clothes and food, being a leaning post.

At 8 am there was a change of shift. The new midwife was called Alma. She was short, with red-orange hair, chirpy. 'It's common to shut down,' she told us. 'Especially if there's been some conflict with the midwife.' She offered to do a trace on the baby's heart so we could go home. The best trace showed that the baby was asleep.

Alma offered us the option of staying in the hospital and sleeping, or going home.

Kate couldn't pooh. She hadn't been since 4 pm yesterday. Alma went to get a prescription for Lactulose. While she was away, Kate did a huge pooh. 'About that long,' she told me. Her fingers were 8 inches apart. The power of Lactulose. Just talking about it makes your bowels move.

Kate was much more alert than I was. The effect of the hormones?

Impossible to sleep with Kate's contractions every six minutes.

Alma was keen for us to go home, to avoid the doctors noticing how long we'd been there. But the difficulty of the transition from home to hospital deterred us from leaving.

She said she'd give us half an hour, but gave us one and a half hours before returning. By then, stronger contractions were back. So we were allowed to stay in the room.

Kate prowled up and down like a panther. She staggered like a boxer in the 15th round.

I ate her lunch. Rice and vegetables.

Six doctors walked in suddenly. They said they wanted to monitor the baby. The earlier trace of its heart wasn't particularly active.

Our midwife, Alma, argued that the baby was just asleep. And she was proved right. The second trace was livelier because the baby was awake. The doctors left. We felt coerced, besieged.

Kate said, 'Bloody hell.'

'What?'

'It's hard work.' Later she said, 'My bum feels weird.'

We received six texts from friends. She didn't want to see them. 'I don't want to know that all these people are waiting for me.'

Kate's waters broke. It happened when Alma was on her break, so it was the supervising midwife who came to examine the discharge on the sanitary towel. She showed it to Kate. 'What colour is that?' asked the midwife.

There was a faint discolouration. 'Green?' said Kate.

Green is the colour of meconium. Baby pooh. A sign that the baby might be in distress. The suspected presence of meconium meant that we wouldn't be allowed to use the birthing pools. But the tinge of green was so pale, it wasn't certain that it was meconium. The midwife went to find a doctor for confirmation.

When a doctor came, Yusuf, he shook my hand. No doctor had done that to us. Yusuf looked at the discharge colour and the trace of the baby's heart and he said it seemed normal to him. He said there was no need for continuous monitoring; intermittent monitoring would be adequate.

So Kate was intermittently strapped to a belt monitor on the bed. The baby's heart rate dropped from 140 to 60 on the graph. I called the midwife. It was because Kate had moved position and the belt was no longer picking up a signal.

2.15 pm. Kate was demoralised, crying, saying she can't go on, worn down by pain.

I was so tired. I sagged at 4.30 pm, but revived after nodding off for ten minutes.

I held the TENS machine while Kate sat on the loo.

Fetching and carrying. During the contractions I kept saying, 'Deep breath in, long breath out, blow it out, blow the pain away, long breath.' I said this about a thousand times.

Kate struggled to find a position that reduced the pain.

At 6 pm a gaggle of doctors came to decide whether to intervene yet. They burst into the room like a gang, like *Reservoir Dogs*. One of them switched on the bright light without asking or warning us. We had dimmed the lights in an effort to make the place more soothing. They watched as Kate leant against me and withstood another contraction, 7.3 on the Richter scale. At this most personal of moments, we are surrounded by strangers. We are on a production line. Stern-faced, the doctors informed us that they would not intervene yet.

Her supper arrived. She said, 'Lovey, you can eat that pie. Not that I recommend it.' Even I wouldn't eat it.

Dan became an uncle recently. It was his sister's first child. Her labour lasted 40 minutes. Now Kate said, 'God, Dan's sister was lucky. Fucking hell.'

A new midwife took over, a young female community midwife, summoned to the hospital 'because they're so busy'.

I was giving Kate Arnica 200 for pain. Aconite 200 for fear and panic. Caullphylum 200 to encourage the contractions.

'You're doing brilliantly,' Kate said to me.

'Thanks, you're doing more brilliantly.'

'I know.'

All afternoon the green tinge on Kate's sanitary pads was suspected of being meconium. But they weren't sure. It could've just been urine.

The new midwife, Mo, was called away. She said that she'd be back soon, but she wasn't.

We spent most of the afternoon without company. In another room, a woman was 29 weeks pregnant with triplets.

Kate refused gas and air. It made her light-headed. 'I don't like the feeling of being drunk.'

During her contractions she watched the second hand on the wall clock. It helped her to get through them.

7 pm. Mo examined the cervix with two fingers. Despite all Kate's hard work, it was only 2 centimetres dilated.

7.20 pm. Kate vomited. Carrots only. Not the peas, interestingly. Mo said it's normal, the body getting ready for labour, getting rid of the things it doesn't want.

7.42 pm. Kate said to Mo, 'Her name's Alice by the way.' It is the first time we have told anybody the name of our baby.

7.50 pm. Kate vomited again.

There was another change of midwives. The new midwife was from central Africa. Nigeria? She read our birth plan. The departing midwife, Mo, who was still in the room, said: 'Have you got a birth plan? Where? I haven't even read it. That's how good I am.'

The new midwife read the section in the birth plan about episiotomies. Kate had written: 'I would prefer to tear rather than have an episiotomy. If an episiotomy is considered necessary by medical staff, we would like to be fully consulted before a decision is made.'

The midwife said, 'It will be a short conversation. Because we will be more concerned with the baby than with your pleasure. There is sometimes a choice between maternal preference and foetal well-being.'

10.20 pm. Kate vomited from gas and air.

10.30 pm. The midwife and two doctors entered the room and sternly informed us that they want to strap Kate to a continuous monitor. All afternoon she had submitted to intermittent monitoring with the approval of the doctor called Yusuf. Now, this gaggle of doctors wanted her to be attached to the machine permanently, restricting her movements. 'It is hospital protocol,' they kept saying, 'when meconium has been found.' This heated discussion was not helping us to establish a comfortable environment for Kate's labour. Yusuf was one of the doctors insisting that we should have been using continuous monitoring since the beginning. This contradicted what he told us before. Clearly he was unwilling to challenge his colleagues. In the end, Kate submitted to continuous monitoring. But we refused a blood test that would leave a needle in her vein. 'I feel like we're being pressurised into a medicalised labour,' Kate told them. So Dr Yusuf consented to defer the blood test and needle.

11.15pm. The doctors reappeared and said that they wanted to see signs of progress. They told us that Kate must dilate at 1 centimetre per hour. Kate was 3.5 centimetres dilated, although the cervix stretches to 4 centimetres.

This seemed crazy to me. The pressure put on the mother to dilate quicker is likely to impede dilation. I'd been trying to make her feel that she's in control, getting what she wants. The doctors' approach was undermining this.

If we ever have another baby, we're not going to the hospital until we can see its head sticking out.

The foetal monitor strapped around the bump kept giving a faulty reading. 'Oh bugger,' said Kate. 'It's picking up my pulse again. Fuck them.'

Tuesday 3 June

12.42 am. Kate said to me, 'Oh, lovey, happy birthday!'

We were swaying, dancing to 'At Last' by Eva Cassidy.

2.15am. Only 4 centimetres dilated.

The Nigerian midwife was sympathetic at Kate's crisis points when she was in extreme pain. The midwife mentioned her own technique for getting through her labour pains: she clutched the bedpost and didn't let go until the baby was out.

At 3.15 am we heard a newborn baby cry in another room.

A couple of times, panting and grimacing after an excruciating contraction, Kate said she couldn't continue any more without the drugs. The first time, I just held her, saying nothing. Then she carried on, forcing herself to breathe through the pain. The next time, when she said that she couldn't carry on, I said: 'You don't have to do anything you don't want to do, lovey.' But she carried on.

The doctors measured the cervix again. By now they wanted to see a dilation of 7 centimetres at least. But it was still only 4 centimetres.

We couldn't believe it. Still trying to breathe through the pain of the contractions, Kate was disheartened. All those hours of suffering and no progress. The continual eagerness of the doctors to intervene. Our fear that a prolonged labour might harm the baby. These things persuaded Kate to agree to be induced.

This meant that an oxytocin drip would be attached to her arm, intensifying and accelerating the contractions and the pain.

She said to me, 'I'm going to have an epidural.' This time there was no uncertainty in her voice. While we waited, she seemed to feel the pain more and more.

It happened at 4 am. The man was like a trainspotter, passionate and knowledgeable about his subject, but not much else. He pushed a needle into her spine.

They advised us to sleep.

She dozed, so I dozed. When I woke up, she was chatting with two midwives. I felt separated from the process. The West Indian midwife was telling Kate that her second child was an epidural. Kate was already swapping epidural stories.

Oxytocin had boosted the contractions up to 'four in ten'. Four contractions in ten minutes.

The midwives were measuring her cervix. They announced that she was 10 centimetres dilated. One hour of a drug had succeeded where 30 hours of contractions had failed. Kate regarded it as a defeat. She felt betrayed by her body.

I brought her some apple juice.

Kate couldn't feel her left leg.

'I want this baby out by a quarter to eight,' joked a young Chinese midwife. That's when the shifts change. 'No pressure.'

They left us alone for an hour. They urged Kate to doze, to conserve her energies for the pushing stage. I was quietly excited. And worried about Kate and the pain ahead.

She was 'fully' at 6.10 am. While Kate dozed again, I heard the Chinese midwife say to the West Indian midwife: 'Head is nice and low. She's feeling the urge to push. The baby is fine.'

When she woke up, Kate wanted to put her contact lenses in, so she could see the baby when it emerged. And to enable the baby to see her eyes. But the Chinese midwife advised her to keep her glasses on for the pushing stage. 'Some people say their eyes popped out,' she said. I assured Kate that the baby will see her eyes.

We were worried about the length of time that Alice had spent in the birth canal. 'She'll have a cone head,' said Kate. She blew heavily through her mouth. She was starting to feel the contractions.

'How you feeling?' asked the Nigerian midwife.

Kate said: 'I feel like I need to pooh.'

'So you haven't missed anything then,' said the midwife. 'That's the urge to push.' Sometimes an epidural can deprive the mother of this feeling.

I had a shave for the baby.

The anaesthetist had told Kate that bonus doses of the epidural were available if she wanted them. All she had to do was push a button on the cord attached to the cannula in her spine. But she was told that if she gave herself a bonus dose in the last half-hour of the labour, it might make the baby dopey. So she resisted the temptation and endured the discomfort as the epidural wore off.

She could feel the contractions but also the pain. She said, 'This is my punishment for enjoying pregnancy so much.'

By a quarter to eight, the baby wasn't out. The change of shift meant that our new midwife was Alma. 'You still here?' she said.

Alma asked, 'Do you mind if a student midwife comes in and observes?' We had stated on the birth plan that we didn't want any students in attendance. We had been warned that they sit in a corner, gossiping.

'How many?' asked Kate.

'Just one.'

'OK.'

The student, Helen, was a nurse retraining to be a midwife. She turned out to be a big help.

What was I feeling? As little as possible. The thought of meeting my baby for the first time brought tears to my eyes. I forced them away. I was here to be useful, not a blubbering mass of tears. I suppressed any feelings. I wasn't in control of anything else, but I could at least be in control of myself.

Kate started to push. And push. And push. She sat and crouched and squatted. She asked for something to bite. Alma and Helen and I supported Kate through two hours of pushing. The baby wouldn't come out.

'Blimey!' said Kate after a particularly harsh contraction. Blimey was an understatement.

Changing position on the bed. Sitting. Squatting. She gripped my hand. I allowed myself to peep down, hoping to see a baby's head, but it was never there. I tried to provide encouragement: 'Pooh it out ... keep going ... big push, go on ...'

'That's it! That's it!' Helen said.

It made Kate think the baby was coming out. 'Can you see it?' she kept asking.

'Not yet,' said Helen, and Kate felt cheated. She thought 'That's it!' meant that the baby was on its way.

Doctors kept appearing at the door. Kate was keen to give birth without their help. Alma fended them off as long as she could.

After two hours, a female doctor came to examine Kate and declared that the baby's head was in the wrong position, hence the lack of progress.

Kate was wheeled to the operating theatre on a bed. Ridiculously, I was told that we couldn't leave anything behind in the room. So I rushed around, stuffing all our things back into our bags. Alma and Helen helped me to carry everything. Suddenly there was a sense of urgency. The slow rhythms of labour were replaced by a mad dash along busy corridors. I had a feeling of disjunction, like an Olympic weightlifter suddenly drafted into a sprint race.

I had to put on a gown, a hat and overshoes. Sheathed in blue cotton, I entered the operating theatre where Kate was trembling on a table surrounded by the surgical team. The anaesthetist didn't acknowledge her, even when administering the anaesthetic. They were preparing her for a Caesarean, just in case. It was ironic that Kate had decided to forgo her final epidural bonus in case the drug affected the baby. Now she was being given a Caesarean-strength epidural anyway. Nothing had gone according to the birth plan.

I wanted to watch my baby enter the world. Instead I bent my head so I could talk into Kate's ear. It seemed more important to be close to her.

She was shuddering, cold, frightened, shocked by the turn of events. I kissed her forehead, which was damp with cold sweat. At first I couldn't speak. Emotions clogged my throat. Now it was my turn to breathe deeply. Then I whispered to her, 'It's OK, lovey. You're in good hands. Our baby will be here soon.' She nodded as tears leaked and dribbled towards her ears. A few moments later, she was speaking with amazing composure.

Bizarrely, the surgeon looked like Sophia Loren. She examined Kate and then calmly reported to us. 'Ventouse isn't an option. I can use forceps to help the baby out. That has a 50:50 chance of success but it would require an episiotomy. Or you can have a Caesarean.'

At first we said Caesarean. Kate didn't fancy having an episiotomy if the chances of success were only 50:50. But the doctor clarified the options. She said that an episiotomy wouldn't be performed unless she was confident that the forceps could do the job successfully. So we gambled on that. We opted to give forceps a chance.

'Any questions?' asked Sophia Loren.

Kate said, 'My friend's baby got a damaged cornea as a result of being delivered with forceps.'

'Your friend was very unlucky,' said the surgeon.

Kate pushed when she was told to.

'Stop,' said Sophia Loren. There was a snipping sound. 'It's going to be OK.'

The forceps, combined with more agonising pushing, got the baby out at the second attempt.

Suddenly the baby was lifted up and placed on Kate's stomach. Crying, covered in blood.

'Oh!' said Kate. She sounded shocked.

'She's OK, she's OK,' I said.

We gazed at our baby. Teary-eyed, I touched her tiny hand with my finger. Remembering my manners, I turned to the surgeon. 'What's your name?' She told me. I didn't take it in. I forgot it instantly. I said, 'Thank you very much.'

'You're welcome,' she said.

Alice was taken into a corner of the room to be examined by one of the paediatricians. We knew this would happen. We had planned that I would follow the baby. But it seemed more important not to abandon Kate. She assured me that she was feeling OK. So I went to see Alice. She scored nine out of ten and then ten out of ten on the Apgar test. She is a healthy baby.

The paediatrician allowed me to cut the umbilical cord, as I had requested on the birth plan. With short scissors I sawed through the sinewy tube. It was only later that I realised that I was at least 10 yards away from Kate. Umbilical cords aren't that long. It had already been cut, of course. They were allowing me a symbolic incision.

I carried the scrawny baby back to Kate on the operating table.

Our baby has hair. We're not sure what colour; it is covered in blood. Big ears. A prominent upper lip. She does look like Charlie Brown. Kate says she is 'pretty, beautiful'.

She was born at 10.44 am. She weighed 7 pounds 7 ounces.

It's my birthday. She is the best gift I've ever had.

INTRODUCTION

Tuesday 3 June (continued)

I carry Alice from the theatre to the recovery room. It is my job to dress her. As I talk to her, explaining what I am doing and apologising for my slowness, I lay her on top of the Babygro and guide her skinny arms into the sleeves. She is tolerant of my clumsiness. She is very alert, with interested eyes rolling hither and thither.

I am snapping the final press-studs together when I notice that something is wrong. The feet of the Babygro are facing backwards. I have put it on back to front. We happen to have brought the only Babygro whose press studs are supposed to be on the rear. I decide that it doesn't matter. It is too long and baggy for her anyway; the foot-shaped sections dangle limply as I carry her back towards her mother.

Kate's bed is wheeled to the William Gillat post-natal ward.

I check my phone. There is a text message from my mum. It says: 'We're on our way.' They haven't actually been invited. I phone her. They are approaching the hospital, having driven 210 miles from Warrington. I tell Kate and Alice that I won't be long. I meet my parents in the car park. My mum is teary-eyed when I tell her that she has a granddaughter. I give them a brief description of the labour and ask them not to question Kate about the details. It is too soon.

Something always happens when I'm away.

Kate is in tears when I return to the ward with my parents. A midwife has changed the baby's nappy. I've missed the moment. Kate wanted to do it herself but the midwife didn't give her the chance.

My parents don't stay long. As they are leaving, two friends arrive. People's faces change when they see the baby. Clare and Nina witness Alice's first burp. They have brought a dog for Alice. Instantly named Patch. Nina cries.

Amazing to think our long-backed girl was inside Kate just a few hours ago. Kate says, astonished: 'Alice was inside me.'

'Yes,' says Nina, 'she looks like something that's been somewhere disgusting.'

Kate's belly still looks as pregnant as ever. We're told it will take six weeks for everything to subside. She is wobbly on her feet and she has a catheter dangling from her vagina. Her temperature goes down to 36°C, then up again.

People gather around Alice as if she's a log fire on a cold day.

She has blue hands and long fingernails, which we're meant to nibble. Her hair is dark, matted with dried blood. She has a forceps mark, a red arc scarring her cheek, which will fade over the next few days.

Some of the midwives give Kate advice about breastfeeding. She is tentative, anxious about picking up her baby. For the first few days, before the milk flows, Kate's breasts will produce a viscous substance called colostrum. Alice sucks this from Kate's finger because she isn't latching onto the breasts properly.

The ward is hot and noisy. From each cubicle comes the flash and whirr of cameras as newborns are surrounded by paparazzi and mamarazzi.

I'm not allowed to stay on the ward past 10 pm. In fact it's 11 pm before I go home. It doesn't feel right to leave them. It is cruel to send a father away from his wife and child on the first night.

I'm weary, unsteady on my feet, as I stagger to the hospital's car park and realise that I can't find the parking ticket. I explain my predicament to the night porter. He asks me how long I have been parked there. I tell him the truth, which seems to surprise him. He says, 'It's £28 but while you've lost your ticket, we'll call it £20.' There is no cash in my wallet. Eventually I find it in my pocket.

Wednesday 4 June

Wake with a jolt after six hours' sleep. I cycle to the hospital and lock my bike to a lamp-post. I am returning to an emotional inferno. Kate is in tears. She had a difficult night on the ward. She went to the toilet and couldn't find her way back to the bed. Someone's baby was crying most of the night. And so was Kate. She had an unsympathetic midwife who was rough with Kate's breasts and who told her not to keep summoning her. 'Pull yourself together,' the midwife told her. A mother from the opposite bed heard Kate crying and came to console her. This mother has been in the post-natal ward for five days after a Caesarean and her baby has an infection; she said that she cried for the first two nights as well.

Kate says her perineum feels like a brick. She isn't in pain but the steps she can make are the length of her foot.

I was so tired last night that I was clumsy, bumping into things, moving and thinking laboriously. Today Kate is the same.

All morning she tries breastfeeding: an ordeal following a trauma following a crisis following torture. And Kate is going through all this without sleep. She hasn't slept for four days.

One of the nicer midwives, Yvonne, stays with us for one and a half hours and helps Kate to breastfeed. Alice is sucking better today, but it's painful for Kate.

Alice has big feet and long toes. I am reflecting that she looks like a grumpy old man, when Kate says, 'She looks like you when she frowns.'

The bumps on her head from birth and forceps have gone down. She looks healthier, bonnier today. She has a habit of latching on to the breast and falling asleep after a few gulps. What the midwives call a 'nipper and napper'.

We phone a few friends. Kate tells her brother: 'It's such a roller coaster of emotions. And she's just sleeping.'

She speaks to her dad. He cries on the phone. 'You're a brave girl,' he says.

One friend asks Kate if she was holding on so that Alice would be born on my birthday. 'God, no, I'd have given anything for her to come the day before.'

I mention to Eddie that Alice was born on my birthday. He informs me: 'You don't look 38. I tell you, you will in a couple of years. Nothing has aged me like being a dad.'

Alice sleeps in a cot next to Kate's bed. The cot is on wheels. We are told to push it to the ultrasound department on the fourth floor. The doctors want to scan Alice's skull to confirm the absence of ventriculomegaly. An Irish doctor declares that her ventricles are 'normal'.

Returning from the ultrasound department, outside the lift, we bump into one of the women from our NHS classes. She hasn't given birth yet. She tells us that her boyfriend has announced that 'he isn't sure if he's going to be around'. I never liked the look of him. I don't know much, but I know this: you can't trust a man who always wears silver trainers. She tells us, 'When he told me what he's been up to, I thought: this isn't what I need two weeks before giving birth.' It is hard to know what to say. We commiserate and say 'Good luck' and walk out of her life.

(Later, I remember a story I should have told her. It's not uncommon for men to panic like this. A friend of a friend, a nice guy, ran away from home a few days after the birth of his first child. After two weeks he returned, talked things over with his wife, and now they are living happily together with their two children.)

When we return to the ward, we get a shock. A doctor tells us that a vaginal swab taken during the labour has revealed that Kate is carrying an infection called Group B Strep. There is a risk that our baby has been infected. This means that Alice will need to be kept in hospital for 48 hours, attached to an antibiotic drip with a needle in her hand. Kate is very upset, crying. She knows of a woman whose baby died from Strep B.

Now our baby must be taken to the fourth floor again. I tell Kate to stay in bed and rest. I travel to the fourth floor with Alice and a male Asian doctor. When the Irish doctor is told about the blood test results, his face falls. He says, 'This is a well baby.' If our baby had caught Group B Strep, she would show symptoms by now. She would have breathing problems; she would be pale; she wouldn't be feeding.

We discuss hospital protocol, clinical judgement. The Irish doctor decides that our baby doesn't need a 48-hour drip after all. There are no symptoms, so he overrules the junior doctor.

In the lift going to the third floor, the Asian doctor explains to me that he is only a junior doctor, lacking the experience of the older man.

When we reach the ward, there is another surprise. Kate has been given a room of her own.

'It's a comedy of errors,' says the young Asian doctor. We offer to move out because our baby doesn't need a drip after all. But they say we can keep the room so I can stay the night.

Kate's Uncle Andrew comes to visit from Oxford. He is a paediatrician. He pushes Alice's big toe backwards until it touches her leg. He hasn't warned us that he is going to do this. He tells us merrily, 'If a baby can do this, there's nothing wrong with its ankle joint.' We hadn't been worried about her ankle joint until he bent it backwards.

The night staff start their shift. The midwife in charge is the one who was rude and aggressive with Kate last night. She comes into our room, accompanied by a junior midwife, to do some routine checks. As they walk out, the senior midwife says to me: 'You can stay until 11 pm.'

I tell Kate to stay in bed. I follow the midwife into the corridor. 'Excuse me?' Her face isn't friendly, but I persevere: 'The day staff told me that I can spend the night here.'

'They had no right to say that.'

'Well, that's not my problem. That's a problem of communication within the hospital.'

Kate hasn't stayed in bed. She comes out of her room to join in the conversation in the corridor. She complains about the way she was treated last night.

The midwife says, 'We're not here to be always sympathetic to the mothers.'

I point out that Kate had endured 38 hours of contractions and hadn't slept for nearly 60 hours. Maybe she deserved a bit of sympathy?

The midwife says that men are never allowed to stay overnight. But I know this rule isn't rigidly enforced. So the midwife tries to enlist the support of her junior colleague. 'It's ward policy. Isn't it?' The junior midwife stares at the floor and nods, not enjoying being put on the spot.

'And,' says the senior midwife, 'there are cultural reasons why men can't be allowed on the ward at night. There are Muslim women on this ward. When men go to the toilet during the night, it upsets the Muslim women.'

'That's fine,' I reply, 'I'll stay in the room. Nobody will see me.'

Faced with determined opposition, the midwife relents and allows me to stay. She even says that I can go to the toilet if I need to. 'What makes me angry,' she says, 'is some men go to the toilet in their underpants.' I promise that I won't do that.

I avoid the toilets anyway. The loos on post-natal ward are used by 50 women dripping blood. The seats are blood-spattered. I tread carefully to avoid stepping on blood-drenched sanitary towels.

Thursday 5 June

At midnight, for the first time I can't stop Alice crying just by talking to her and holding her. This isn't so pleasant, when she's crying incessantly, beyond my influence. Only a breast would calm her down.

Kate winces when Alice bites her nipple. But she won't ask for help from the midwives on the night shift because they were so nasty last night.

Alice feeds for a full hour until 1 am, the best yet. When breastfeeding goes well, we're all happy. Then Alice does her biggest ever pooh, a lake of sticky meconium. The novelty of nappy-changing is wearing off already.

In the morning, Alice has her first bath. A black midwife shows us how to do it. We've been helped by so many people. Nine out of ten midwives are fantastic. It's just the odd one that's a witch.

'Wicked witches and fairy godmothers' is Kate's assessment of the umpteen midwives we've seen.

At 10 am we go to a breastfeeding workshop run by Yvonne. Alice and Kate are still finding it tricky. Alice wouldn't latch on this morning. In the waiting room we spoke to several mothers who shared their annoyingly efficient birth stories. One woman, whose baby boy was born early this morning, said her labour lasted 2 hours and 50 minutes and her baby is breastfeeding keenly already. 'He won't stop!' She was 9 centimetres dilated when she arrived at the hospital. She had one significant advantage. She's 18 years old.

When Yvonne turns up, she asks us to introduce ourselves. I am the only male there who is more than a week old. I say, 'I'm Alice's dad.'

Yvonne laughs and turns to Kate. 'You've been demoted. He used to be Kate's partner and now he's Alice's dad.'

After the breastfeeding workshop, I go shopping at Camberwell Green for maternity pads and paracetamol. Cycling makes me realise how exhausted I am. Slow-minded with fatigue, I have to think about everything twice.

In the afternoon there is another breastfeeding workshop. When I arrive, I find Yvonne manually squeezing drops of milk out of Kate's breast. We will have to express milk and feed Alice from a cup until she learns to latch on to the breast properly.

Kate has been finding expressing difficult because of the problem of collecting the milk in a plastic cup as it trickles under her breast. She also got frustrated with cup-feeding; some precious colostrum tipped onto Alice's chin.

Yvonne says to me: 'Do you think you could do this?'

This request comes as a surprise, but I'm here to be as helpful as I can. I pretend to be delighted. 'At last I'm allowed to touch them!' Yvonne teaches me the painstaking technique. I have to put a thumb and finger on either side of the areola and feel for the milk ducts; they're like grains of rice under the skin. Then my fingers press down and eek a few drops of milk out of Kate's nipple. I scoop each drop into a small plastic cup as it trickles over Kate's broad brown areola. I am milking her.

Alice has been dopey all day, sleepy and apathetic. Her eyes roll behind her lids. She isn't the energetic baby I knew yesterday. When we mention this to Yvonne, she suggests that we ask someone on the ward to test Alice's blood sugar levels. This involves pricking her foot with a needle and collecting a smear of the blood on a test-strip. Alice is so lacklustre now that she doesn't flinch when the needle pierces her heel.

The result is low: 2.3 instead of 2.8 or 3.0.

This confirms that Alice isn't getting enough food. Now it's vital to express more colostrum from Kate's battered breasts. I find the milk ducts on either side of her areola, press them in and squeeze together for three seconds and colostrum seeps out of two or three places in the centre of the nipple.

This afternoon she expresses a couple of millimetres. This evening we manage to express another millimetre, which I cup-feed to Alice by supporting her head and tilting the small plastic cup against her lower lip; she sticks out her tongue and she laps up the liquid. A few drops are left in the cup. We're not supposed to waste a drop, so we have to dilute this colostrum with sterilised water so she can drink it. But I am tired and stupid. Unthinkingly, I put tap water in there. Babies aren't allowed to drink tap water. Precious drops of colostrum have been squandered.

Then we are told not to feed her again until the next blood sugar test at 6.30 pm. If Alice's blood sugar is high enough, we'll be allowed to go home.

Until then we must carry on expressing colostrum. Lots of tears from Kate. We are, both of us, exhausted and worried. At least she gets meals from the hospital. I am living on the chocolate birthday cake that Clare and Nina gave me. There is no time to rest or visit the hospital's café. Even though she hasn't slept for several days, Kate's mind is hyperactive. I am constantly performing little tasks.

Alice wakes up. Her eyes are bright and alert again.

But the next blood sugar level is 1.5. This means we won't be going home today. The evening test is 1.7.

I cup-feed Alice a couple of times with breast milk donated by Kate.

Feeding Alice is one of the nicest things I've ever done. Her face is pretty now that the forceps marks are fading; her head is small and round with pale-brown/dark-blonde hair; she looks like a little bird as she laps the breast milk.

We go upstairs to the special care baby unit for paediatric assessment. More blood tests. The level is 2.8 now thanks to Kate's concentrated expressing and feeding during the evening.

Blood is taken from Alice's right hand. She cries and gives the doctor a dirty look.

A doctor tries to persuade us to use formula milk. She tells Kate that 'it's not a failure' if you can't breastfeed your baby. But we are determined to keep trying, knowing that breast milk is better for the baby. In the end they agree to give us a 60ml container of donated breast milk. But tomorrow, they say, we'll have to use formula milk.

Friday 6 June

Alice sleeps on my chest until 4 am. Then Kate tries to breastfeed her. Alice does her usual trick of latching on, sucking for a few seconds, then lying there inertly. After ten minutes, as advised by the midwife on duty, I warm up the donated breast milk. Alice has a dramatic sense of timing. At this exact moment, Kate says: 'She's learnt how to do it!' Alice stays attached and sucking for 17 minutes, her longest feed yet. It is a great, uplifting moment. I feel suddenly awake and optimistic again. 'It's a roller coaster,' says Kate.

Afterwards, to compensate for her depressed fontanelle and dehydrated skin, we cup-feed Alice the donated breast milk as well. The midwife finishes the cup-feeding for me; Alice is falling asleep and I am too gentle to wake her up.

Then we all try to get some sleep. Alice's blood sugar levels will be tested before and after each feed. Until her blood sugar level is higher than 3.0 on 2 consecutive tests, after being fed solely by Kate, we won't be allowed home.

Blood sugar level at 7.15 am after a feed: 3.7!

Blood sugar level at 8.45 am before a feed: 2.9.

When we feed her at 9 am, she is a lazy sucker again. Kate is anxious about the competence of her breasts. 'I feel as if my tits are on trial,' she says.

Finally, after feeding and expressing colostrum, Kate sleeps. I feed Alice with the cup. Then I have to fetch things from home and Mothercare.

While I'm absent, a Caribbean midwife comes and takes Alice away for a blood sugar test. When she returns, her tone is severe and critical. 'It is 2.1!' the midwife complains to Kate. 'This baby has not been getting a feed!'

After Kate tells me this story, I protest to this midwife that her comments aren't fair or helpful. If all the midwives were one person, they would be treated for personality disorder because of their fluctuating moods and manner. We never know what kind of person is going to walk through the door.

Two point one? We are shocked that the reading is so low after Alice fed for so long on Kate's breast and I cup-fed her some expressed colostrum.

The Caribbean midwife weighs the baby. At birth Alice weighed 3.390 kilos. Today, after 4 days, she weighs 3.040 kilos. A difference of 0.350 grammes. Babies often lose 10 per cent of birth weight in the first few days. Our baby has lost 10.3 per cent. This slight difference means the midwife will inform the paediatrician. He will insist that the baby must be weighed every day. I'm starting to think they'll never let us go home.

Kate notices in the medical notes that it says 'baby's weight loss greater than 10 per cent'. It doesn't say *slightly* greater. It doesn't say 10.3 per cent.

The wards are hot. Several midwives have told us not to put too many clothes on Alice, and the breastfeeding tutors encourage skin-to-skin contact. Now the Caribbean midwife tells us to put more clothes on her so that she won't get cold and lose more weight.

They contradict each other and they contradict themselves. The Caribbean midwife instructs us to feed Alice in three hours. As she is leaving the room, she says we can feed Alice immediately if she is hungry.

Kate gets really hot while breastfeeding. I use a small battery-powered fan to cool her down, directing it towards her face and neck. I never direct the fan at the baby. But the Caribbean midwife has written in our medical notes: 'Dad is using a handheld fan on mother and baby even though advised to keep baby warm.'

We are constantly surveyed and tested to see if we're doing things in a way they approve of. One of the galling aspects of parenthood is that you get treated like a child.

Kate is tense. There is strain in her face, anxiety in her voice. She smiles at people and it is an expression of pain.

Alice falls asleep on my chest. It's such a pleasure being a mattress for her, giving her warmth and comfort. I feel as if I'm doing something useful, and I get to lie down at the same time.

This is a unique moment. Alice is asleep and, briefly, we are giving Kate's breasts a rest. We decide to look at the cards that people have sent us – I brought them from home for Kate to see. While she is reading them out loud, I fall asleep. Then Kate falls asleep. We lie in comas for an hour.

She phones friends who've had babies. Some of them have endured similar ordeals in the first days after birth.

Kathy comes to the hospital. She sits with Kate while I go home for more things that Kate wants, such as clean clothes and the radio–cassette player, things that I took home three days ago, thinking we were about to leave hospital.

As Kathy is still breastfeeding her twins, she generously offers to donate some of her breast milk to Alice, but the suggestion is rejected by members of staff because her milk hasn't been screened.

Then a midwife brings four bottles of breast milk to Kate, specially granted from the hospital's supply of donated milk. One of them, containing 40ml of milk, has already been warmed so it has to be used within the hour. It is a bottle with a teat on it.

Some midwives have advised us not to use teats if we want to breastfeed. Babies get confused. Now we're confused.

Kate phones me at home, where I am packing things she wants. I can hear Alice screaming in the background. The desperation in Kate's voice makes me agree to use the teat. I cycle back to the hospital and feed Alice with it. A deeply satisfying experience. Her small face and big eyes are full of expressions.

Things are getting better. Then they get worse. The Asian doctor, whose name is Janak, comes to tell us that one of Alice's blood tests has revealed a high CRP score. I don't know what a CRP score is, but I can tell it isn't good news.

'How high?' I ask.

'Eighteen.'

'How high should it be?'

'About five.'

So we return to the special care unit on the fourth floor. A doctor called Amit tells us that a high CRP score might indicate that the baby is fighting an infection. Amit wants to insert a cannula in Alice's hand so that antibiotics can be inserted twice a day.

Kate doesn't want to watch. She stays in the corridor. But the chairs are too hard for a woman with an episiotomy, so she goes back to the ward. I stay with Alice in the intensive care unit, watching tiny babies in incubators.

Amit sticks a needle in Alice's hand. She pulls a face, but doesn't wake up. Then Amit is beeped on his pager and he goes away. 'Won't be long,' he says. He doesn't come back for half an hour. I stand next to the intensive care cot where Alice is lying under a hot lamp. Her head glistens with sweat. I notice a sign on the intensive care cot. 'To avoid the effects of over-heating, do not leave a baby unattended.' I bring the sign to the attention of a nurse and she lowers the heat. Amit comes back, slightly flustered. There was an emergency with another baby. He straps a cannula into Alice's hand and a nurse gives her a first dose of antibiotics.

The irony is that we elected to give Alice an oral dose of vitamin K to spare her the pain of an injection. She's had 50 injections for blood tests already.

The doses of antibiotic will be administered twice a day. It's my job to wheel the cot to the special care ward at 6 am and 6 pm at least until Monday. Then we should get the results of the cultures, hopefully confirming that she hasn't got an infection. If she has? God knows how long we'll be stuck here.

I've told Alice, 'Life isn't always like this. It gets better.'

Kate's breasts are sore but functioning. The colostrum is thinner, paler, becoming more milky. Now we need Alice to learn how to use the breast efficiently so we can leave this place.

Kate is frantic. Her mind is restless, racing from thought to thought. Most tasks she can't do herself, so she asks me. Every time I sit down, she thinks of something else. For me, today was another day without rest or a proper meal.

Saturday 7 June

We feed Alice until 2.45 am. I sleep in the reclining chair that has a habit of unreclining with tremendous force. It's like an ejector seat. After a short feed at 5.15 am, on breast and bottle, I take Alice upstairs for infusions of antibiotics from a South African nurse.

Downstairs I attempt to sleep again, but we end up trying to get Alice to feed. She is reluctant to suck the breast – she has become used to the teat in recent feeds. She is suffering from 'nipple confusion' says a tall, calm African midwife. 'The important thing is not to give up.'

Alice coughs up milk twice this morning, once all over her Babygro when the African nurse is watching. She advises me to wind Alice more regularly. So I'm adding that to the routine.

In fact, I've been forgetting to wind her at all. I'm an idiot.

'Take a picture?' suggests Kate. So I pick up the camera to take a picture of her and Alice. 'I'm starving!' she complains, as if I am forcing her to stand there for a photo, as if this was my idea. Kate leaps from thought to thought, task to task, anxiety to anxiety, in a second. The problem is that her mind is going at 100mph and mine, deprived of sleep and female hormones, is going at 2mph.

This morning I cycle home for an uninterrupted sleep lasting an hour and 50 minutes.

People don't know we're still in the hospital. There is a message from Craig on the answerphone at home. He says, 'I hope I'm not disturbing your peace ...'

I'm trying not to be irritated by Kate's irritability. She has had 6 or 7 hours sleep during the last 100 hours. I'm in the hospital 99 per cent of the time, but 1 per cent of the time I'm at home or shopping for urgent supplies. I can walk out of the situation, but she can't. That 1 per cent is worth a lot.

A woman tries to leave the ward with her baby. Police bring them back. The baby is on the child protection register. Now the mother is only allowed to visit the baby while sitting behind the reception desk where the midwives can keep an eye on her.

Another blood sugar test: 2.6.

Kate says that 'breastfeeding is a really nice feeling'. It makes her feel relaxed and drowsy. Then Alice bites her nipple and she yelps.

More friends come to visit. Sophie describes Alice as 'an objectively pretty baby'. When Kate tells the story of the birth, Nina has to leave the room.

When there are moments to think, I can't help going over the events when we arrived in the hospital, especially the reception from the midwife who tried to dissuade Kate from using the birthing pool. I was out of the room, bringing our luggage. I feel bad that I couldn't stop it happening. This midwife made the hospital seem uncomfortable and unwelcoming and unsupportive. 'She froze my labour,' says Kate.

People say they're going to visit for five minutes, then stay for an hour because Alice is so lovely. They get excited when she opens her eyes or pulls one of her faces. Some friends are a great support. Other friends aren't so helpful. Tara turns up and says, 'What a nice room!' She is missing the point. To us it feels like a cell.

The paediatrician we don't like is Cindy. Today she says: 'We'll weigh her tomorrow and if she hasn't put weight on we'll have to think again.' Which just puts more pressure on Kate to perform.

I go to the special care ward at 6.30 pm for Alice's blood test. Then she is given antibiotics. We return an hour later for another blood test; they are assessing the levels of antibiotic in her blood.

The test involves pricking Alice's heel with a needle. At first she won't bleed enough because her foot isn't warm, so she is pricked again. The nurse squeezes her foot to force the blood out. She fills two short straws with Alice's blood. She says Alice is a pretty baby. 'I've never known a baby with such strong legs,' says the nurse. Alice ends up with her head at the top end of the cot from wriggling and protesting so much. Her little feet are bruised from all these needles.

At 8.30 pm it finally happens. Kate feels tired and feverish. This is one of the signs that her milk is arriving. She lies back on the bed to sleep for a while. While she dozes, I feed Alice with the thin yellow colostrum that Kate has already expressed. Alice drinks all 30 millilitres, having already fed from Kate's right breast. Afterwards we sit together. I straighten her back and rub her spine. The first burps are gratifying.

She is perched on my lap when her face grimaces. I hear a squelch and feel a plop against my leg. I sneak a look. This isn't sticky meconium. It is Alice's first proper nappy: fulsome, brown, viscous and quite smelly. I feel happy. It is a pleasure to be shat on.

It takes me a while to clear the mess up. Some of it has run up her back because the chair seat slopes backwards. After I've changed her nappy, a midwife happens to come in. She looks at Kate, zonked out on the bed. The midwife tells her to drink lots of ice water to help the milk fever to pass. She urges Kate to allow Alice to feed off her breasts to stop them becoming engorged.

Alice feeds again. This is the most she has consumed during these first five days. She has discovered her appetite. It feels as though a crisis has passed.

I stare at her and feel lucky. It feels like a privilege to have this little person in our lives. She is delightful. Full of expressions.

A second pooh-filled nappy follows an hour after the first.

Sunday 8 June
One of the midwives arrives at 4 am for a pre-feed test of Alice's blood sugar. The result is 4.3. The midwife is pleased for us. 'What have you been feeding her, cake?'

Kate has been working hard, feeding and expressing from both breasts. Our next trial is to show a weight gain when Alice is weighed today.

Alice cries and grumbles half the night. We cuddle her, but she is inconsolable. We think it is the new pressures inside her body. While sleeping in bed with Kate, she has a pooh of such proportions that we have to change the bed sheets.

Amidst the tyranny of feeding, Kate asks me: 'When are we ever going to sleep?' She is laughing, but it is a real concern for us.

My plan to doze in the chair for a couple of hours is thwarted by Alice waking at 5 am. I carry her up and down the room to stop her disturbing Kate. At 6 am I take her to the special care ward for antibiotics. The nurse looks at her leg tag and keeps calling her Kate.

What little sleep I'm getting is always interrupted by a crisis. I doze from 9 until 12 when Kate shakes my leg. She can't wake Alice up, so she has decided to wake me up instead. She is desperate to feed Alice before she is weighed. So I run cold water over my hands and apologise to Alice for the disturbance. I wiggle her legs, open her Babygro and put my cool hands on her skin. It doesn't work. In the end, giving her a wash wakes her up.

At lunch, the dinner lady kindly leaves us two meals, so I can eat one too.

Kate is in pain. 'I feel like I've got a rock up my bottom.' Her nipples are sore. Sometimes she winces when Alice is feeding. 'I want to go home,' she says. We have a policy now of only saying positive things when staff ask us questions.

Cindy asks us how much the baby is eating.

How are we supposed to know that? The problem with breasts is that there's no gauge to measure how many millilitres of milk are being dispensed. Kate makes up a figure. 'Forty millilitres per feed.'

Cindy seems satisfied and leaves, saying that she won't weigh the baby today after all. She'll weigh her tomorrow instead.

We're at the mercy of the medical mathematicians.

Alice is feeding well today, but she still isn't keen on the right breast. Unfortunately, Kate doesn't feel able to ask the midwives for help in case they write something in her notes that extends her confinement in hospital. We have a nice new hospital room, but it feels like a prison.

Kate's granny is pleased that we're still stuck in hospital. 'Good,' she said when she heard the news. She thinks that new mothers are sent home too early these days. In her day, all new mothers and babies stayed in hospital for two weeks.

The friends who visited yesterday are here again. We invited them back because yesterday's visit was so gloomy.

Sophie says that, based on her experiences, whatever we do won't be good enough for the hospital staff. Her daughter was below average weight so the doctors wanted her to go on formula feed. Later her daughter was above average weight, so the doctors again wanted her to go on formula feed.

In St Thomas' Hospital, Jack was told off for carrying his newborn baby. 'You might drop him,' said a nurse. The hospital policy was to wheel babies around on trolleys. Jack ignored them.

These stories cheer us up. Midwives and doctors don't tell us these things. They just make us feel that we're failing if our baby isn't conforming to the stipulated weights and measures in their textbooks. Talking to friends is a source not only of sympathy but also of alternative information, challenging the health professionals' rigid version of baby development.

I tell them about Amit, the doctor in the special care unit, who told me that he would keep all newborns away from strangers for 28 days to avoid risks of infection.

I ask Jack if he has any tips for waking up a sleeping baby. He says, 'Try to get some sleep yourself.'

We find an envelope that our friends have left behind for Kate. It contains a cheque for Kate to treat herself when she's free.

Monday 9 June

Alice feeds until 1 am, then lets us sleep. At 6 am I take her to the special care ward for antibiotics. In the lift and in the corridor, everyone smiles when they see her. Back in our room, I sleep till 10.30 am.

With the help of Fybrogel, Kate has had a couple of poohs and is feeling better. It has released some of the pain, she reports.

Today we're waiting for Alice's latest CRP score. One of the midwives warns us that another baby with a high CRP score had to stay in hospital for two weeks.

Someone has nicked the lights screwed to my bike. It makes me think of the old joke: 'We are here to help others – what the others are here for, I don't know.' I cycle home. Kate wants me to send some photos to relatives. I email a digital photo to friends and family: the one of Alice, seven hours after birth, perched on Kate's tummy next to a huge breast. Kate has given me permission to send this.

While I am at home, Kate phones to tell me that 'Alice has been weighed and she has put on 200 grammes in the last two days, which is brilliant'. Babies aren't expected to regain their birth weight until the second or fourth week, and Alice is well on the way already. The pressure they put on us was excessive.

Alice has been feeding relentlessly all day and Kate's breasts are spurting milk. She has to massage the hard parts. Her perineum is still sore; the most difficult part of breastfeeding now is sitting down.

Kate's milk is starting to flow like Niagara. One midwife advises her not to express too much milk in case her breasts became engorged and she contracts mastitis. (This well-intentioned but erroneous advice had serious consequences. Her milk production declined. Getting it back was hard work. With sleepy babies, we've read since then, it's wise to encourage milk production by expressing after feeding.)

Friends have given Kate a rubber ring to sit on. It is the first time I've seen Kate smile since the beginning of contractions. It eases the pain in her sore areas. But one of the midwives has noticed the ring. 'You're not sitting on that, are you?' She says it makes blood fill the perineal area and delays healing. It's better to sit with your thighs raised on rolled-up towels.

The evening's midwife is a lovely Irishwoman called Carmel. She sees me giving Alice some expressed breast milk in a bottle and says, 'Can I give you a tip? I hope you won't be offended. It's better to cup-feed than to bottle-feed, to avoid nipple confusion.'

We smile and tell her that we agree, but we've been advised and pressured by other midwives who've instructed us to use teats rather than cups. Teats teach babies a different sucking motion and make them lazy because it's easier to extract the milk from a teat than a nipple. To prove the point, Alice spews a mouthful of breast milk that she hasn't been able to digest.

'You're lucky they didn't come in and whisk her away and give her a formula feed,' says Carmel. She is sympathetic. She says, 'Trust your instincts as parents.'

'We'll go home, then,' I reply.

We are supposed to get Alice's blood culture results today. If they give her the all-clear, confirming that she hasn't got any infection, we are hoping to be allowed to go home.

But we are told this evening that the results have failed to arrive. We are also informed that even when the antibiotics are withdrawn, Alice will have to remain in hospital for 24 hours for observation in case she has an allergic reaction to the build-up of antibiotics in her system. This means we can't go home until Wednesday at the earliest. We are prisoners of the hospital.

Tuesday 10 June

A doctor visits us from the special care ward. She says, 'Did you get my message yesterday? I phoned down about 1.30 in the afternoon to say the results wouldn't be ready.'

'We weren't told until the evening,' says Kate.

'Oh, I'm sorry. We've got the results now and they're negative, so we can stop the antibiotics. If there ever was anything there, we've got rid of it. How is baby?'

'Very well.'

'Is she feeding well?'

'Yes.'

'She looks well. Normally we insist on a 24-hour observation period after antibiotics, but if she's still looking fine this evening, we'll let you go home.'

That's the good news. Now the bad news.

Kate tells the tall African midwife, Mabel, that her perineum still feels sore. The last person to examine it was the abrupt Caribbean midwife who glanced at Kate's vagina and declared that everything was fine. Mabel now examines her vagina more conscientiously and announces that one of the stitches has come loose. Later a doctor comes to look at it. The loose stitch means that Kate's cervix might take longer to heal.

One of my cousins in Warrington, Kim, was at work when she received the photo that I emailed to family and friends. She printed it to show her colleagues. Embarrassed by the breast, she cut it out of the picture before showing the photo around the office.

Kate has a new trick. She stands over the sink and shows me proudly how milk squirts out of her 2-inch nipples. She squirts Alice in the eye. 'Oh sorry!'

Things are calming down. Kate can walk rather than shuffle. She manages to sleep this afternoon while Alice dozes peacefully in her cot. I have lunch in the hospital canteen.

When Kate wakes from her afternoon nap, feverish and sweaty, she asks me to take Alice off her breast and put her in the cot. I point out that she is already in her cot. Kate looks at me as if I am stupid. I am stupid, but on this particular occasion, I am right. Kate looks into the cot and sees Alice there. She looks down at her breasts. 'I could feel her there,' she says. 'Maybe this is what Kathy meant about going mad when she started breastfeeding.'

The paediatrician wants us to wait until the evening to make sure that Alice shows no adverse reactions to the antibiotics. Her temperature mustn't go above 37 degrees. The nice Irish midwife, Carmel, takes her temperature in the early afternoon. She stares at the thermometer.

'Is it all right?' asks Kate.

'It's 37.1,' says Carmel. 'No, hang on.' She is counting the dots on a plastic strip as they change. 'It's 36.7. That's OK.'

I cycle home to tidy up. Dishes from seven days ago. A week's dust. I resist the temptation to lie down, just in case I lapse into a coma. I haven't slept in a bed for a week. I drive back to the hospital.

As I carry bags and towels and a radio–cassette machine out of the maternity ward, I look as if I am returning from the beach. The midwife sitting at the desk glances at me and says: 'The holiday's over.'

I carry Alice out of the hospital. The sun is shining. Sitting in the car is painful for Kate. I try to avoid the speed bumps. Alice cries as she enters the flat. She can only be consoled by her mother's breast.

We sleep.

Babies are born without bony kneecaps. I didn't know this. Kneecaps don't ossify until a child reaches two to six years of age. There are many surprises among the marvels of gestation and growth. A baby has 300 bones. But an adult has only 206 bones. Many bones, such as those comprising the skull and spine, fuse together as we grow. Teeth are the first thing to decay while we're alive and yet the last thing to decay when we're dead.

Of the 75 trillion cells in the body, about half of them are red blood cells. Each red blood cell contains about 250 million molecules of the iron-containing protein called haemoglobin, which is capable of picking up four molecules of oxygen. As a result, a single red blood cell can deliver up to 1 billion molecules of oxygen. Laid end-to-end, the arteries, capillaries and veins would stretch for about 60,000 miles in the average child and would be about 100,000 miles in an adult – enough to wrap around the world nearly four times. A nose can distinguish up to 10,000 different smells. (Mine can't.) The tongue has 10,000 taste buds. The mouth produces about 1.7 litres of saliva each day; over a lifetime, that's enough to fill two swimming pools. The adult brain contains 100 billion neurons – more than the number of stars in the Milky Way galaxy. Each of the brain's neurons connects to as many as 100,000 other neurons. At 3 pounds, the brain makes up only 2 per cent of total body weight but consumes 25 per cent of the energy used by the entire body. In one day, the brain is able to process 86 million bits of information. (Mine isn't.) Each lens in the eye is made up of 22,000 fine layers of transparent cells stacked in rows like crystalline bricks. The retina has 125 million rods and cones. The human eye can detect differences between nearly 8 million different shades and colours. The ear can discriminate between more than 300,000 tones. The inner ear has 20,000 hair cells, each with 100 separate hairs (2 million in total), each responding to its own frequency and intensity of sound. The human head contains 22 bones. More than half of your body's bones are in your hands and feet. The hand is a wonder of engineering. With its 27 bones, opposable thumb, unique fingerprints and flexibility, a hand can perform a multitude of complex tasks. Hand skin is tough enough to withstand considerable abuse, yet sensitive enough to feel the lightest personal touch. There are 72 feet of nerve fibres in the hand. If all our nerves were stretched out in a straight line, it would be 45 miles long. Each square inch of skin contains as many as 650 sweat glands, 20 blood vessels, more than 1,000 nerve endings and has up to 20 million bacteria on its surface. The average man has about 20 square feet of skin weighing about 10 pounds. The face has 28 paper-thin subcutaneous muscles, which move skin rather than bone, allowing us to make 250,000 facial expressions. In one day, the average person takes between 8,000 and 10,000 steps. Has 103,689 heartbeats. Breathes 23,040 times. Moves 750 major muscles. Speaks 48,000 words. Sweats up to 12 litres of water. Sheds about 45 hairs. Casts off 600,000 particles of skin each hour. The average three-year-old has two pints of blood in their body; the average adult at least five times that amount. The human body contains about 36 litres, or 8 gallons, of water. Your heart pumps more than 6 litres of blood every minute, nearly 10,000 litres a day. In one day, your blood travels nearly 12,000 miles. Your heart beats around 35 million times per year, about 3 billion times in an average person's lifetime, pumping a million barrels of blood – enough to fill three supertankers.

And all this began as a fertilised egg cell smaller than the head of a pin. Our baby didn't have an easy task. It's astonishing that anybody is born wholly healthy and intact.

Pregnancy, like aerial bombardment, produces feelings of shock and awe. Is it worth it? Yes, it is. A baby restores your sense of wonder. I've seen the Himalayas and the Grand Canyon. Nothing is more impressive than my baby's smile.

Despite all the emotional turmoil and practical chaos, parenthood is an orientating experience. It feeds a need to devote myself to something worthwhile. It is more satisfying than a Ferrari.

Money is the most important of life's least important things. I still haven't got much. I am supposed to be a provider. What can I provide? I will try to provide love. Kate is a very loving person. Our baby won't be short of that.

In the lonely moments of my life, I've missed loving as much as I've missed being loved. Love is something we create as well as consume. That's why we say that we make love; we don't say that we take it. Love is best as a conversation, not a monologue. Alice has joined our conversation and taken it in new directions.

Having a child makes you more conscious of, and connected to, the fundamentals of life, of birth and being. It is a bittersweet experience. Not just because of the laboriousness of caregiving. In gaining so much, we are conscious that we also have more to lose.

Our offspring has sprung. Her life has begun. The hard part is over. Now the difficult part begins. We are entering what Naomi Wolf, cheerful as ever, calls the fourth trimester: 'the sometimes savagely difficult adjustment period that follows birth'.

There are no happy endings. In the end we all die. I am just grateful that Alice's story has, at least, a happy beginning.

Now it's time to change a nappy. The book stops here.

to my daughter
to my wife
to my mum
to my gran